MODERN DRUG DELIVERY SYSTEM: INNOVATION AND APPLICATION

By Dr. Ashish Srivastava

- Chapter 1: Introduction To Drug Delivery Systems: History And Significance 3
- Chapter 2: Principles Of Pharmacokinetics And Pharmacodynamics In Drug Delivery 8
- Chapter 3: Nanotechnology In Drug Delivery: A Revolutionary Approach 15
- Chapter 4: Liposomes And Micelles – Targeted Drug Carriers 24
- Chapter 5- Transdermal Drug Delivery: Non-Invasive Methods And Techniques 33
- Chapter 6: Oral Delivery Systems: Advances And Limitations 42
- Chapter 7: Ocular Drug Delivery: Targeting Eye Diseases 50
- Chapter: 8 Pulmonary Drug Delivery: Treating Respiratory Conditions 57
- Chapter 9 Injectable Drug Delivery Systems: Improving Patient Compliance 65
- Chapter 10 Controlled-Release Systems: Improving Therapeutic Outcomes 74
- Chapter 11 Polymers In Drug Delivery: Enhancing Drug Efficacy And Stability 83
- Chapter 12- Biodegradable Systems: The Future Of Sustainable Drug Delivery 92
- Chapter 13: Gene Therapy And Viral Vectors: Innovative Drug Delivery Solutions 101
- Chapter 14: Regulatory Challenges In Drug Delivery System Development 110
- Chapter 15 Future Perspectives: Emerging Trends And Technologies In Drug Delivery 118

Chapter 1: Introduction To Drug Delivery Systems: History And Significance

Drug delivery systems have existed as part of medicine for thousands of years. The concepts, however, used now are much different than in yesteryear. The concept of the introduction of therapeutic agents into definite sites in the body finds its roots way back in the ancient civilizations in which they used herbal remedies, tinctures, and other forms of early poultices to heal several aliments. The last few decades, however, have seen a completely new approach that has developed drug delivery techniques at a highly rapid pace to acquire precision in therapy while trying to enhance the patient experience and outcome.

1.1 Drug Delivery Evolutions

Drug delivery began with primitive routes such as oral and topical applications that relied upon the available natural chemicals that could control the amount and concentration. These early methods, although relatively effective, lacked specificity, thus creating side effects and ununiformed results. It wasn't until the pharmaceutical revolution in the 20th century that better controlled methods of drug delivery were produced. Synthetic chemistry allowed the researcher to formulate drugs of increased potency and specificity; from this beginning, the modern delivery system was able to be born. To achieve a prolongation of drug concentrations in the bloodstream for extended periods, controlled-release formulations were developed. The systems represented a paradigmatic shift in that they provided predictable and sustained drug release to avoid the pitfalls of variable drug levels and frequent dosing. Techniques like encapsulation in capsules and hydrogels and polymers led to the formulation of drugs, which could be administered systematically, thus revolutionizing patient management of chronic diseases such as diabetes, hypertension, and cancer.

1.2 Role of Drug Delivery Systems in Contemporary Medicine

Unless there is an efficient delivery system, no therapeutic drug can be successful in a contemporary medical setting. Enhance the absorption efficiency of drugs, increase compliance, reduce side effects, and allow drugs to target specific tissues-all these objectives are beneficial for patients and pharmaceutical companies looking to enhance the therapeutic values of their products. For example, a better delivery system makes a compound with poor solubility and absorption become a most effective therapeutic drug.

A drug delivery system, therefore plays a vital role in a long-term therapeutic treatment process of conditions like cancer, HIV, cardiovascular diseases, or chronic inflammatory conditions. It can bring about targeted delivery into diseased tissues and help minimize drugs' exposure to healthy cells, thereby avoiding adverse effects. These are particularly useful in oncology, where precise delivery and minimal off-target effects are critical due to the cytotoxic nature of most chemotherapy drugs. Minimizing drug exposure to healthy cells reduces side effects, thereby allowing for a direct tumor site delivery at a higher dose and maximizing the treatment's overall effectiveness.

1.3 Types of Drug Delivery System

As diversified as the diseases they promise to treat, today's drug delivery systems are. There are the main types comprising the scope of this text:

Oral Delivery Systems: The oldest and certainly by far the most traditional is the oral route. A tablet, capsule, and liquid are absorbed through the gastrointestinal tract but pose problems in bioavailability-except for drugs broken down by digestive enzymes or with the poor absorption of drugs.

Injectable Systems: Injections enable drugs to be introduced through needles into the bloodstream directly in the body. It finds widespread use in vaccines and insulin and other therapy when drug concentration needs to be very tightly controlled.

Transdermal Systems: Transdermal patches are systems created to deliver drugs via human skin. This application avoids the gastrointestinal tract by delivery of drugs and can administer sustained release over a definite period.

The Inhaled Systems: These types of drug delivery systems suit people with respiratory diseases such as asthma, COPD, and infections. Targeting the lungs directly maximizes the delivery and effectivity of drugs used on them.

Targeted Delivery Systems: Using nanotechnology, the system delivers targeted cells or tissues, targeting molecular sites, such as on cancer cells, ensuring lower collateral damage and resulting in better therapeutic outcomes.

Gene Therapy and Viral Vectors: These advanced delivery systems involve modifications of viruses or other delivery systems to introduce genetic material into cells, which hold promise for therapies in genetic diseases and some cancers.

Controlled-Release Systems: These systems are engineered to release drugs at a controlled rate to maintain therapeutic drug levels within the body for an extended period with fewer injections, thereby enhancing patient compliance.

1.4 Challenges and Future Perspectives

Developing drug delivery systems is not easy; from compatibility with a variety of drugs to the regulatory pathway, it encounters many challenges. For instance, developing a drug carrier that would deliver a therapy effectively yet nontoxic and biocompatible requires a lot of research and testing. Another challenge for the pharmaceutical industry is to make these systems available and inexpensive for patients.

Despite all these challenges, the future of drug delivery holds promise. The emerging technologies include personalized medicine, which would tailor therapies to individual patients based on genetic, environmental, and lifestyle factors, thus transforming drug delivery. Personalized delivery systems are likely to improve treatment efficacy and reduce side effects as drug release patterns are adjusted according to the unique physiological profile of each patient.

The next exciting frontier would be artificial intelligence in drug delivery. Artificial intelligence could potentially speed up the discovery of novel drug carriers, optimize dosing regimens, and predict the response of patients to drugs. In the near future, AI-driven models may even enable real-time adjustment of drug release to further improve treatment outcomes.

Chapter 2: Principles Of Pharmacokinetics And Pharmacodynamics In Drug Delivery

A great working knowledge of Pharmacokinetics and pharmacodynamics is essential in drug development and optimization in terms of drug delivery. PK provides insight into the mechanisms where drugs are absorbed, metabolized, distributed, and excreted within a biological system, whereas pharmacodynamics focuses on drug-activity interactions with biological and biochemical targets within target areas of the body.

2.1 Understanding Pharmacokinetics: Process of ADME

ADME is the four main processes involved in pharmacokinetics: Absorption, Distribution, Metabolism, and Excretion. All these processes determine the drug concentration in the bloodstream, which subsequently determines its availability at target sites. There are unique challenges and considerations that each stage poses for designing drug delivery.

Absorption- Absorption is the process by which a drug enters the bloodstream from its site of administration. The main absorption site of orally administered drugs is the gastrointestinal tract but happens to pose certain difficulties in terms of digestive enzymes, pH levels, and the intestinal barrier. Drug delivery systems should take into account these factors to increase bioavailability-that is, the amount of drug that reaches the bloodstream in its unchanged form. Many advanced delivery techniques, including enteric coatings and nanoparticles, are used to ensure the increase in stability of drugs in the process of absorption.

Distribution: Drugs get circulated in the body through entering the bloodstream, to achieve their target tissues. Some factors that affect the process of distribution include blood flow, tissue permeability, and protein binding. A good delivery system should ensure a drug reaches its target location in a way that exposure of the rest of the tissues results in unwanted side effects.

Metabolism: The metabolism of drugs generally involves the participation of enzymes, which, primarily in the liver, may convert the drugs into either active or inactive substances. This may significantly affect the drug's efficacy and the duration for which the drug would exert its effect. Avoidance or circumventing substantial metabolism by drug delivery systems can enhance the effectiveness of drugs. In transdermal and inhalable delivery systems, avoiding first-pass metabolism through the liver, more active substance of the drug would reach the target site.

Excretion: Finally, the drugs and their metabolites are eliminated from the body through the excretion system, mainly the kidneys. The rate of excretion affects the half-life of the drug or the period that it is active in the body. Long-acting systems usually result in slow release of the drug to prolong the duration of action of the drug and consequently reduce the dosing frequency.

2.2 Pharmacodynamics: Mechanisms of Drug Action

The science of drug-receptor interaction in the body that pharmacodynamics describes is really concerned with how drugs produce their therapeutic effect and can also cause adverse effects due to their interference with endogenous substances. For a good delivery system of drugs, a balance needs to be struck between achieving the utmost possible therapeutic effect and side effects need to be at a minimum.

Binding on specific receptors- Many drugs activate through binding on specific receptors on the outer surfaces of cells, whether activating or blocking to ultimately produce a physiological response. One example is targeted drug delivery systems using antibodies or molecular ligands to bind precisely to the receptors on the diseased cells and exclude binding on healthy cells; receptor specificity, therefore, avoids side effects and increases the level of therapy.

Dose-response Relationship: Dose response defines the relationship between the drug's dosage and its effect to give the best possible dosages. Drug delivery systems would control the rate at which a drug is released into a system, and ideally such a concentration must lie in the therapeutic window-when its effect can be clinically recognized but the concentration remains well below toxic values. Thus, controlled release or sustained release systems are created that hold such a balance where there is the steady release of drugs through time.

Therapeutic Index: The therapeutic index refers to the measure of drug safety, which is computed as the ratio of toxic dose to the therapeutic dose. Drugs with narrow therapeutic indexes require very tight blood concentration control to avoid toxicity. Drug delivery systems are particularly valuable for drugs that have narrow therapeutic windows as they help maintain consistent levels within the therapeutic range, and controlled-release and targeted systems are especially valuable.

2.3 Challenges in Drug Delivery: Biological Barriers

One of the major challenges in drug delivery is to overcome barriers set up by the body that protect it against foreign bodies-substances, including drugs. Effective treatment can only be achieved if delivery systems can be designed to effectively pass through these barriers.

Blood Brain Barrriers: BBB is a cellular protective barrier that keeps the brain safe from some possibly harmful substances found in blood. However, this has been a significant restraint in delivering drugs to the brain for neurological diseases like Alzheimer's and Parkinson's diseases. Now days the researcher includes nanoparticles and liposomes for safely crosssing through blood brain barriers and carrrying drugs to the brain.

GI Tract: The main challenges posed to orally administered drugs by the GI tract include the following: acidic pH of stomach, digestive enzymes, and intestines with varying absorption rates. The enteric coat or encapsulation in liposomes can be used in order to avoid the degradative effect of acid in the stomach on the drug preparation and thus stabilize and make the drug absorbable at the GI tract.

Cellular Barriers: The drugs must traverse cell membranes at the cellular level to reach their site of action. Hydrophobic drugs can diffuse readily across the membranes, but hydrophilic drugs cannot pass through cell walls. Methods employed for cell uptake include nanoparticles and conjugation with lipid carriers.

2.4 Role of PK/PD in the Design of the Drug Delivery System

Design of drug delivery systems based on a pharmacokinetic and pharmacodynamics understanding leads to optimal therapeutic outcomes. The following list some of the major ways through which PK/PD principles guide drug delivery.

Optimization of Bioavailability: Drug delivery systems ensure that maximum amount of drugs reach the systemic circulation of blood. This is achieved by such formulation of nanoparticles, micelles, and lipid-based carriers in order to protect the drugs from degradation and enhance the absorption and bioavailability process.

Improving Stability of Drugs: Many drugs, mostly biologics and proteins, are very sensitive to environment conditions like temperature and pH. Encapsulation in polymers or liposomes stabilizes such drugs, sustaining their activity for longer periods.

Protraction of Drug Action-It is possible to increase the duration of action for the drug by controlling its rate of release, wherein an implant or extended release formulation can prolong the activity of a drug, leading to less frequent dosing and improved patient compliance.

Reducing side effects-When applied directly to the site of action, this reduces the exposure that the rest of the tissues has to the drug with less side effects. There are targeted systems like in the case of antibody drug conjugates, where this will deliver drugs to disease cells precisely, allowing doses at the target area in much higher quantities than by sparing healthy cells.

Improving Patient compliance-It is easier to improve compliance in patients since non-invasive forms of drug delivery, such as a transdermal patch or an inhaler, are very acceptable to the patients, so that the treatment regimen adopted turns out to be the correct one. These are applied extensively in chronic conditions needing a long-term therapy cycle.

2.5 Case Studies: PK/PD in Action

Many of the successful drug delivery systems that are in use today result from the impact of PK/PD principles. The following are two examples of where PK/PD optimization has significantly improved treatment outcomes:

Diabetes and insulin pumps: Fluctuations of blood glucose levels will often occur in the case of traditional insulin injections. Insulin pumps provide a controlled and steady delivery of insulin throughout the day, mimicking the natural response of the body to insulin delivery. PK/PD information enhances the blood glucose control and reduces complications.

Liposomal Doxorubicin for Cancer: Doxorubicin is an extremely effective chemotherapeutic agent having toxic effects on normal tissue. Encapsulation of the agent within the liposomes further ensures drug targeting to only tumor cells. This eliminates much exposure to normal tissue and would eliminate cardiotoxicity as well as adverse side effects to allow its better usage as a safety means of anticancer agent.

Chapter 3: Nanotechnology In Drug Delivery: A Revolutionary Approach

One of the most revolutionary breakthroughs in modern drug delivery is nanotechnology. It allows the engineerings of extremely small versatile carriers called nanoparticles through which drugs can be delivered with an unprecedented precision. Such particles fall in the size range from 1 to 100 nanometers. It provides several advantages of using it in medicine including the increased targeting, controlled drug release, and improved solubility for drugs of low bioavailability.

3.1 The Basics of Nanotechnology in Medicine

Nanotechnology in drug delivery is the development of particles that can deliver drugs to target cells or tissues in the body. Nanoparticles, due to their small size, could possibly cross biological barriers, like the blood-brain barrier, which prevents entry into the CNS. More importantly, nanoparticles can be made to interact with the diseased cells, targeting therapy, thereby sparing the healthy cells and reducing the side effects.

Other aspects of nanotechnology are multiple options of drug delivery, which are liposomes, dendrimers, micelles, and polymeric nanoparticles among others. Each category provides a unique characteristic best suited for various therapeutic treatments-from cancer drugs to gene therapy. Therefore, the multiplicity in nanoparticles has remained at the center of various research studies and developments related to drug delivery systems.

3.2 Classifications of Nanoparticles in Drug Delivery

There are several kinds of nanoparticles used in drug delivery. Each has a combination of properties that suit the application.

Liposomes: Liposomes are spherical vesicles with a lipid bilayer that can encapsulate hydrophilic (water-soluble) drugs, as well as lipophilic (fat-soluble) drugs. This structure closely resembles a cell membrane, which favors good compatibility and uptake into the target cells. Therefore, liposomes are among the most commonly used vesicular systems in cancer therapies because drugs can be delivered specifically to sites of tumors while evading side effects on surrounding tissues.

Polymer nanoparticles: It include the biodegradable polymers through which the drugs get release in controlled rates. Many times, polymeric nanoparticles are used for sustaining the release of drugs from these drugs. This elongates the time of therapeutic window for the drug. Their applications come in such chronic diseases whose levels of drugs need to be maintained. Their merits arise more when, in the case of these diseases, they provide the needed drugs levels, so, hence, in cardiovascular or in diabetic disorders, their employment is relatively easy.

Dendrimers: A branched tree-like molecule which features a highly large area surface for attaching drugs makes it an excellent source. With the property of highly ordered structures, high capabilities to exactly load followed by the accurate drug release qualify them as being ideal candidates for targeted drug delivery. Due to its highly proficient ability towards functionalization, applications in gene therapy have very recently been sought after for targeting delivery purposes across the blood-brain barrier.

Micelles: These are spherical nanoparticles formed from amphiphilic molecules that contain both hydrophilic and hydrophobic properties. They are specifically useful in delivering poorly water-soluble drugs, as the hydrophobic core of the micelles can encapsulate such drugs, increasing their solubility and bioavailability.

Metal nanoparticles: Gold and silver nanoparticles exhibit some distinct properties like ease of functionalization and optical responsiveness, making them suitable for diagnostic imaging and photothermal therapy. They can be designed to deliver drugs on demand based on the response to external stimuli, such as light or heat.

3.3 Mechanisms of Drug Release and Targeting
The mechanisms of drug release are engineered into nanoparticles, and specificity to targeted locations is achieved in drug delivery by enabling specificity in the nanoparticles.

Control Release: The goal of controlled-release nanoparticles is to prolong the length of time during which drugs are available within the body to achieve therapeutic levels. Controlled-release particles are particularly useful in conditions where frequent dosing is inconvenient or where steady drug levels are needed. Using pH-sensitive or temperature-sensitive materials, nanoparticles can be designed to release drugs in response to specific triggers, such as an acidic environment of a tumor.

Targeted Ligands: The targeting ligands attached to the surface of nanoparticles include such moieties as antibodies or peptides. These ligands interact with specific receptors on target cells, thus ensuring the drug will only be received by diseased cells with minimal exposure to healthy tissues. Targeted drug delivery is widely applied in the area of cancer therapy, with nanoparticles being used to administer chemotherapy drugs directly to the cells within the tumor and reducing the toxicity while at the same time enhancing the efficacy of the therapy.

Stimulation responsive release: nanoparticles could be designed to respond selectively to particular stimuli like changes in pH, enzymes, light, or magnetic fields. The pH-sensitive nanoparticle has the drug payload, releasing it when there's a low pH; they could be applied directly against tumour cells that mostly live in low-pH regions. Some could even deliver drugs with the presence of infrared light so drugs may only come out upon non-invasive, demand-release orders.

3.4 Applications of Nanotechnology in Drug Delivery

Due to their capabilities, nanoparticles have been widely applied in various therapeutic fields.

Cancer Therapy: The most exciting application of nanotechnology can be seen in drug delivery for cancer therapy. Conventional chemotherapy drugs are toxic not only to the targeted cells but also to normal tissue, resulting in a broad range of side effects. It is possible to deliver such drugs directly to the cancerous site by using the nanoparticles and reducing the impact of side effects so that higher doses of the same drugs can be administered to the patient. The present two nanotechnology-based applications of cancer treatment that can be used in clinics include liposomal doxorubicin and nanoparticle albumin-bound paclitaxel.

Nanotechnology has given hopes to the treatment of neurological diseases such as Alzheimer's and Parkinson's and brain tumor. Nanoparticles help to pass through the blood-brain barrier, hence not being able to penetrate a number of drugs to reach the brain. The focus on research on liposomes, polymeric nanoparticles, and dendrimers for targeting the therapeutic agents to CNS gives an opportunity to come up with more effective neurodegenerative disease treatment.

Gene Therapy: This is a method to effectively deliver genetic material - like DNA or RNA, as a nanoparticle delivery form - directly to the target cells. This directly strikes at the root of disease. Traditionally, the choice for gene delivery is based on viral vectors; however, they pose inherent concerns about safety. Researchers and scientists are looking towards nanoparticle carriers that include non-viral forms of carriers such as liposomes and dendrimers that hold promise for cystic fibrosis, muscular dystrophy, and certain cancers therapies.

Infectious Diseases: Nanotechnology has shown potential in treating infection by amplifying the efficacy of antibiotic and antifungal medications. The nanoparticles can release antimicrobial agents directly to the infection site, hence increasing their effectiveness and making it unlikely to develop resistance. Vaccine development is another application of nanoparticles. Currently, researchers have been performing studies on mRNA vaccines related to COVID-19 using lipid nanoparticles for efficient delivery.

Cardiovascular Disease: Nanoparticles can be targeted to atherosclerotic plaques of cardiovascular diseases. Nanoparticles could potentially reduce heart attacks and strokes by locally delivering anti-inflammatory drugs or clot-dissolving agents directly to plaque sites. For instance, polymer-based nanoparticles may release drugs at a controlled rate at the site of plaque, which will decrease the need for highly invasive procedures.

3.5 Case Studies: Nanotechnology in Clinical Practice

Many nanotechnology-based drug delivery systems have gained clinical application and are already useful in practice for the improvement of outcomes for patients.

Liposomal Doxorubicin (Doxil®): This is doxorubicin in its liposomal form, administratively used to treat most types of cancers, both breast and ovarian. As it is encased by the liposome, more nontoxic drug stays within the drug and diminishes the level of cardotoxicity along with most of the adverse effects towards other healthy tissues. Being targeted by a liposome allows the drugs to release its effects maximally only to the tumors.

Abraxane® (Albumin-Bound Paclitaxel): The chemotherapy drug paclitaxel, which is widely used today as an intravenous agent in many medical conditions, suffers from its poor solubility in water, reducing the effective concentration of bioavailability at the tumor sites. Albumin nanoparticles of paclitaxel significantly increased the solubility, thus enabling much higher dose levels to achieve high, therapeutic concentrations. It's particularly successful with metastatic breast cancer and pancreatic carcinoma, as well as advanced non-small cell lung carcinoma, as the first systemic therapy for this aggressive cancer is significantly less toxic compared with conventional formulations of the chemotherapeutic.

m RNA COVID-19 Vaccines (Pfizer-BioNTech and Moderna): Success of these recent mRNA vaccines relies upon lipid nanoparticles carrying mRNA coding for the spike protein from SARS-CoV-2. Particles offer protection to such fragile m RNA and ease its cellular entry where cells instruct immune systems to work upon such viruses and, thus produce antibodies. Hence, development of COVID 19 Vaccines is done in quite a rapid but effective way due to critical importance that lipid nanoparticle delivery holds.

3.6 Future Directions in Nanotechnology for Drug Delivery

Nanotechnology for drug delivery is a bright future since continuous research on novel types of nanoparticles and novel mechanisms for delivery is being carried out.

Personalized nanomedicine: Nanotechnology will allow drug delivery systems to be designed for specific genetic and physiological characteristics at the individual level. For example, personalized nanomedicine may one day change how treatment is approached by taking into consideration the best delivery approach for each person.

Smart Nanoparticles: Researchers are developing "smart" nanoparticles that could sense its environment or respond to diverse stimuli. Some smart nanoparticles change phase from hydrophobic to hydrophilic at one temperature, for instance, so drugs can be delivered more precisely.

Hybrid Nanoparticles: This could make possible multifunctional systems by integrating the features of different types of nanoparticles. Hybrid nanoparticles with a combination of magnetic and polymeric properties are developed for combined imaging and therapy, which allows doctors to monitor real-time drug delivery.

Biodegradable Nanoparticles: Nanoparticles that degrade naturally in the body reduce the chance of toxicity and accumulation. More and more biodegradable materials, such as polymers and lipids, are being used so that nanoparticles leave no trace after their therapeutic task is accomplished.

Chapter 4: Liposomes And Micelles – Targeted Drug Carriers

Liposomes and micelles are the most potent drug carriers based on nanoparticles. Their unique structures and properties make them ideal for targeted delivery of drugs directly to their target sites, thus avoiding side effects and enhancing the therapeutic outcome. These are especially useful in oncology, neurology, and infectious disease treatment, in which targeted delivery is considered to be essential in preventing adverse effects on healthy tissues.

4.1 Liposomes and Their Functionality

For example, liposomes are spherical vesicles that have the structure of cell membranes; they are characterized by one or more layers of lipid bilayers that surround an aqueous core. Liposomes can carry both hydrophilic (water-soluble) and hydrophobic (fat-soluble) drugs.

Biocompatibility: Liposomes are made of either natural or synthetic lipids, and they are biologically compatible. They can be engineered to avoid the immune system, which increases the circulation time of the drug in the blood.

Drug Loading Capacity: The structure of liposomes allows the encapsulation of a wide range of drugs. A hydrophobic lipid bilayer may encapsulate fat-soluble drugs, while an aqueous core may encapsulate water-soluble drugs. Therefore, flexibility for multi-drug therapy is presented here.

Controlled Release: Liposomes can be designed to provide drug delivery in a controlled and sustained manner, giving a long-term therapeutic effect. By modulating the lipid composition, drugs release at a set rate to provide for instant delivery and controlled prolonged delivery.

4.2 Types of Liposomes and Their Applications

Liposomes can be categorized depending upon the structure, size, and surface modification of the liposomes. Several types of liposomes exist due to differences in advantages that a specific type of liposome offers for various medical applications.

Traditional Liposomes: These are the least sophisticated liposomes, prepared with phospholipid and cholesterol. These have primarily been used for release systems, though they tend to be rapidly cleared from the circulation by the immune system. They can be useful in applications in which exposure to the drug for a temporary period is acceptable.

Stealth Liposomes Stealth liposomes are coated with polyethylene glycol that hides them from the immune system. This "stealth" effect prolongs circulation time so that the liposomes can reach more distant or difficult-to-access target sites, such as tumors. Stealth liposomes are used in the treatment of cancer by directly delivering drugs like doxorubicin to tumor cells

Cationic Liposomes: Positively charged. Used where negatively charged membranes are of concern. Extremely useful when employed in the context of gene therapy - to simply drive DNA or RNA molecules straight into cells; used also to carry mRNA or genetic material in a vaccine to administer.

pH-Sensitive Liposomes: These liposomes release their drug payload in response to acidic environments, such as in tumors or infection sites. The pH-sensitive feature enables targeted drug release specifically at diseased sites, thus minimizing exposure to healthy tissue.

4.3 Mechanisms of Drug Delivery and Release with Liposomes

Liposomes deliver drugs mainly through two mechanisms: fusion with cell membranes and endocytosis. Understanding these mechanisms helps in designing effective liposome-based drug delivery systems.

Fusing with Cell Membranes: Certain types of liposomes fuse with cell membranes. Their content is thus delivered directly inside the cell, as for drugs acting within the cell, for instance certain kinds of anticancer and antibiotics medications.

Endocytosis: Besides that, liposomes also enter the cells through the process of endocytosis. Here, cell membrane engulfs liposomes and brings them inside to break it inside the cell by releasing the drug. Its function is particularly good for transferring genetic material and protein-based drugs.

4.4 Summary of Micelles and Functions

Micelles are another type of nanoparticle used in drug delivery. These are particularly used for drugs that are hydrophobic and have low water solubility. Amphiphilic molecules are those which possess both hydrophilic as well as hydrophobic regions. This special arrangement enables micelles to hold hydrophobic drugs inside their core, thus increasing the solubility and bioavailability of the drug.

Self-Assembling Structure: Micelles spontaneously assemble as soon as amphiphilic molecules are introduced to the aqueous environment; with hydrophobic domains arranging themselves together to make the core, and hydrophilic domains on the exterior surface. This self-assembled nature makes micelles so easy to prepare and offers great flexibility in terms of drug encapsulation.

High Solubility of Poor-Solubility Hydrophobic Drugs: The hydrophobic core contains micelles. Thus, low-solubility drugs are enclosed into the hydrophobic core of the micelle so that the solubility and, therefore its absorption in the body becomes better. This property is of help especially for the hydrophobic cancer drugs

Stability: The Micelles are stable in blood circulation and do not provide conditions for the degradation of payload drug. This type of stability allows the longer retention of the micelle within the blood, thereby enhancing the possibility of successful drug delivery at the required target site.

4.5 Classification of Micelles and their Application

Micelles are classified on the basis of molecular level structure, surface modification, and stimulus response. There are various types of micelles that exist to serve the purpose of different drug delivery.

Polymeric Micelles

Polymer-based micelles are derived from synthetic polymers that are highly stable and can be circulated for a relatively longer period. Polymeric micelles are mainly used in cancer therapy for the delivery of insoluble chemotherapeutic agents.

Mixed Micelles: These micelles are a mixture of various amphiphilic molecules, which enables the encapsulation of several drugs or the stabilization of a drug. Mixed micelles can be formulated for combination therapy, in which two or more drugs are administered together to achieve enhanced therapeutic effect.

Stimuli-Responsive Micelles: These are the kinds of micelles that will respond to the drug stimulus with specific triggers, such as temperature, pH, or enzymes. They can be of great utility for targeted delivery of drugs and emptied appropriately in specific sites, such as at the acidic environment of the tumors.

4.6 Applications of Liposomes and Micelles in Medicine

Liposomes and micelles are very much used in broad therapeutic fields, from tumor therapy to infectious diseases to many other applications. Both liposomes and micelles can be excellent methods for targeting drugs and tailoring their release profiles and, hence, are valued tools in modern medicine.

Liposomes and micelles-based nanoparticles are highly used in oncology, especially for enhancing the chemotherapy drug delivery. The formation of the drug within such nanosystems decreases the harmful effects of the formulation towards the healthy tissues; however, it increases its concentration at the tumor area. Liposomal doxorubicin and paclitaxel-loaded micelles are few of the nanoparticle based formulations used in cancerous treatments.

Infections: Liposomes and micelles have proven to be useful in infectious diseases because they enhance the delivery of antimicrobial agents. Amphotericin B, being an antifungal agent, is incorporated into formulations in the form of liposomes, thus reducing toxicity and increasing the efficacy of the drug. Micelles are also used for antiviral drug delivery and improve their stability and solubility.

Neurological Disorders: The treatment of neurological diseases is difficult because the BBB restricts drugs from entering the brain. Liposomes and micelles can be engineered to bypass the BBB, where the drug can be targeted at Alzheimer's and Parkinson's disease. Scientists have recently been working on liposome-based nanoparticles that have been engineered to carry drugs to traverse the BBB for diseases that are specific to certain conditions.

Gene Therapy: Both liposomes and micelles are used in gene therapy for the delivery of genetic material. Liposomes, especially cationic liposomes, can be used to encapsulate DNA or RNA, protecting it from degradation in the bloodstream. Micelles are also being studied as non-viral vectors for gene delivery, which is safer than the traditional viral methods.

4.7 Case Studies: Clinical Success of Liposomes and Micelles

Doxil® (Liposomal Doxorubicin): Doxil is one of the best known liposomal formulations that are used in cancer treatment. Liposomal encapsulation of doxorubicin has significantly reduced its cardiotoxicity, which is the major side effect of the conventional drug doxorubicin, and enhances the delivery of the drug to tumor cells. Doxil has been successful in treating ovarian cancer and Kaposi's sarcoma among other malignancies and, therefore, represents clinical success of liposomal drug delivery.

AmBisome® (Liposomal Amphotericin B): AmBisome is a preparation of the antifungal drug, amphotericin B, in which the active ingredient is given in liposomes. Thus, encapsulation in a liposome reduces the inherent nephrotoxicity of this drug, significantly reducing one of the major severe side effects of conventional preparations of amphotericin B. AmBisome has improved the management of a number of patients with various types of invasive fungal infection, especially for immunocompromised subjects.

Genexol®-PM (Paclitaxel-Loaded Micelles): Genexol-PM represents a micellar formulation of paclitaxel used in cancer therapy. Encapsulation in a micelle increases the solubility of paclitaxel, thus significantly reducing its dependence on poisonous solvents and improving consequently the therapeutic efficacy of this drug. Genexol-PM is most usefully applied in breast, lung, and ovarian cancer.

4.8 Future Directions for Liposomes and Micelles

The future of liposome and micelle research lies in increasing targeting specificity, enhancing drug loading capacity, and building stimuli-responsive systems for even more precise drug release.

Multifunctional Liposomes and Micelles: A single delivery system that can provide combination therapy through the ability of liposomes and micelles to carry multiple drugs or therapeutic agents. Multifunctional systems can target different pathways of diseases such as cancers with improved treatment outcomes.

Smart liposomes and micelles. Stimulus-responsive smart nanoparticles which will respond to various stimuli that include temperature, pH levels, and levels of some enzymes are an attractive concept. Such systems are predicted to provide an ability of precise control of the drugs' release only when reached the target site.

Hybrid Nanoparticles: Mixing the liposomes' and micelles' features with another nanoparticle may provide other characteristics like those of gold or magnetic particles to result in designing hybrid imaging and therapeutic systems. Hybrid nanoparticles could also serve for real-time monitoring of the drug delivery to ensure patients can be followed on treatment plans.

Chapter 5- Transdermal Drug Delivery: Non-Invasive Methods And Techniques

Transdermal drug delivery is an almost entirely non-invasive and patient-friendly method of delivering drugs. It goes through the skin directly into the bloodstream as opposed to some conventional administration routes that go via orals and injection where GI Tract and Hepatic metabolism are circumvented and consequently provide controlled, slow releases of drugs for over extended durations. The current chapter is directed towards dealing with the mechanism, type, benefit and limitation of Transdermal drug delivery system applications with future direction.

5.1. Mechanisms of Transdermal Drug Delivery

The skin is basically designed to protect the body from harmful substances. Because of this, delivering drugs through the skin is challenging. Drug delivery systems should cross this barrier but control the drug release into the bloodstream. The first step toward this end is to know the skin structure:

Skin Structure: There are three significant layers that the skin contains, such as the epidermis, dermis, and hypodermis. The most superficial is the stratum corneum, and because of this dense keratinocytes with lipids in the makeup, this area is permeation resistant; thus drugs have to traverse this.

Drug Permeation Mechanisms: Drug transport in a transdermal system basically depends upon the diffusion, which in many cases may be carried through the dermal layer; there is the following transdermal route:

Transcellular Pathway: Transcellular pathways basically need drugs for crossing from cell to another; however the drugs with higher solubility is required in order to gain entry.

Intercellular Pathway: The drugs diffuse between the skin cells. This is a general pathway for hydrophilic molecules.

Follicular and Sweat Gland Pathway: This route uses hair follicles and sweat glands. In this route, molecules may take the shortcut into the skin.

The physicochemical properties of the drug like molecular size, lipophilicity, and solubility affect its penetration into the skin. Smaller, more lipophilic molecules are generally penetrated better and used in transdermal delivery.

5.2. Classes of Transdermal Delivery Systems

Transdermal drug delivery systems fall into various categories, each with a distinct profile, advantages, and utility.

Transdermal Patches: They are the most common delivery devices; transdermal drug delivery systems are adhesive patches in composition. These patches generally are designed to have layers in multiples for controlling release rates over time. Such patch types include:

Reservoir Patches: Composed of a gel or liquid drug reservoir, with an invariant rate of drug delivery.

Matrix Patches: The drug is carried within a polymer matrix which allows for controlled, sustained diffusion.

Multilayer Patches: It can also be used in the multilayer form for tough formulations of drugs. It might be used in combination as a treatment for complicated diseases. Topical Gels, Creams, and Ointments: These types of formulations are used primarily as localized treatments, but some systemic effects are possible if used on certain areas of the body, such as on the skin. As such, they are suitable drugs that require quick release because they are easy to administer.

Microneedle Patches: These are patches that have very tiny, painless needles that create microchannels in the skin, so larger molecules, such as vaccines or hormones, can be delivered effectively. This is an emerging technology that has shown promise in immunization and therapeutic peptide delivery.

Iontophoresion and Sonophoresion: These are advanced techniques that use external energy sources to enhance drug permeation through the skin:

Iontophoresis: It applies a mild electrical current to push charged drug molecules into the skin so that the dosage and the timing can be controlled.
Sonophoresis: The ultrasound waves are used in this method to temporarily damage the stratum corneum, which is the most outer layer of the skin so that it becomes more permeable to drugs.

5.3. Advantages of Transdermal Drug Delivery

Transdermal drug delivery offers several advantages over the other methods. This is why some types of drugs are particularly suited for transdermal drug delivery:

Non-Invasive and Easy to Administer: It is painless and not invasive, which makes it comfortable for the patient and improves patient compliance.

Controlled Drug Release and Steady Levels: The transdermal drug delivery systems can release the drug at a controlled rate, hence providing consistent therapeutic effects. It maintains steady blood levels as opposed to peaks and troughs that may cause side effects or decreased efficacy.

This bypasses first-pass metabolism and the acidic GI tract. Drugs given transdermally directly enter systemic circulation without needing to go through the liver or having to be exposed to the acidic GI environment. Therefore, drugs given transdermally have higher bioavailability and a higher percentage of the drug can reach the target site.

Improved Patient Compliance: Transdermal systems do not demand frequent dosing, which is an advantage for patients suffering from chronic conditions. For example, a weekly hormone patch can replace daily pills or injections.

5.4. Limitations and Challenges

Even though transdermal drug delivery has so many benefits, there are still many challenges and limitations that exist.

- The main limitation of the skin's barrier function is that the range of drugs that can be delivered effectively is quite limited. Only drugs having physicochemical properties, including small molecular size, moderate lipophilicity, and non-ionic, penetrate the skin efficiently.

- The potential for skin irritation and allergic reactions from prolonged exposure to transdermal patches or adhesives may pose a limitation to their use in some patients. Such a reaction may be a cause for concern, especially for sensitive individuals.

- **Drug Loading Capacity**: The volume of drug a transdermal system can carry is limited, which might prove to be a limitation for those drugs that require high dose levels to be effective.
- **Absorption Variability**: The thickness of the skin, hydration level, and temperature are all different in different individuals, so the rate of absorption will vary. For example, in warmer conditions, the blood flow to the skin is increased, which may facilitate the absorption of drugs in a faster rate.

5.5. Transdermal Drug Delivery Applications

Transdermal drug delivery is used in many therapeutic fields, mainly in those conditions which demand steady and long-term dosing.

- Hormone Replacement Therapy (HRT): Estrogen and testosterone are often administered through transdermal patches in a controlled release manner for stable hormone levels; side effects from oral hormone therapy are prevented.

- Pain Control: Transdermal patches filled with analgesics such as fentanyl control the pain of chronic and cancer patients. They effectively decrease the frequency of oral doses while limiting the risks of taking oral opioids.

- Nicotine Replacement Therapy: Nicotine replacement by nicotine patches controls a regulated amount of nicotine so that the patient is encouraged to quit smoking as they progressively reduce their nicotine intake.

- Nitroglycerin patches are administered for the treatment of angina to ensure that a steady dose of nitroglycerin is delivered to the body, thereby preventing angina attacks from occurring.

- Vaccine Delivery. Microneedle patches are promising for delivery in vaccinations when small, precise quantities are needed. Such microneedle patches will also be ideal for mass immunizations since they do not need refrigeration and can easily be administered.

5.6. Advanced Technologies in Transdermal Drug Delivery

Over the years, it has been possible to have additional capabilities of transdermal systems beyond the original ones of patches and creams.

- **Electroporation:** This is the process involving short electrical pulses that induce transient pores in the skin. Thus, larger molecules such as peptides or proteins penetrate easily.

- **Microneedle Arrays for Biologics:** Microneedles are now designed to deliver biologic drugs which normally cannot cross the skin. Arrays of dissolvable microneedles made of biocompatible materials are an innovative method of vaccine and therapeutic protein administration.

- **Transdermal Wearable Devices**: Advanced devices are in development combining transdermal delivery and sensor monitoring wearables, which may be able to maintain a constant flow of biomarker monitoring- such as glucose or electrolytes in the case of diabetes-and closed-looped adjustment of transdermal drug delivery with real-time treatment.

7. Emerging Trends and Future Directions

- Transdermal drug delivery continues to advance, providing future technologies and trends: more versatility, more efficient delivery, or both.

- Future systems will likely respond to biological signals, such as blood sugar levels, releasing drugs when they are most needed. For instance, a bioresponsive insulin patch could deliver insulin in proportion to increasing blood glucose levels.

Polymeric and Biodegradable Patches: Research is currently under way to create degradable patches made from polymers. The degradable patches would not have a major environmental impact and also do not harm the patients.

- Nanotechnology integration: Using nanoparticles is the current focus of investigation for carrier-based permeation enhancement across the skin. Nanoparticles will feature as encapsulation agents to provide future generation transdermal products with better stability and tissue targeting.

- Combination Therapy Patches: A patch containing several drugs could improve therapy in such complex diseases as cardiovascular disease or chronic pain. In such diseases, a combination therapy patch might be formulated with delivery of both the pain reliever and an anti-inflammatory so that there would be a proper delivery of pain control.

Conclusion

Transdermal drug delivery is indeed a marvelous approach in medicine these days that provides a secure, comfortable, and pain-free method for the slow release and controlled delivery of drugs. The application of this drug in different uses, such as pain management, hormone therapy, smoking cessation, and vaccine delivery, shows its promise. However, the natural barrier function of the skin presents a barrier to transdermal delivery; hence, formulation techniques and delivery technologies are continually advancing through research and innovation. Combining technology advancements in wearable systems, bioresponsive patches, and microneedles, the future of transdermal drug delivery holds high promise for expanding treatment options and improving patient compliance across a wide array of medical conditions.

Chapter 6: Oral Delivery Systems: Advances And Limitations

The most commonly accepted route of administration is oral drug delivery, which allows convenience, ease of use, and generally good patient compliance. However, despite these advantages, oral delivery systems have a few challenges: limited absorption, enzymatic degradation, and first-pass metabolism, which may significantly influence the bioavailability and efficacy of drugs. The book reviews the modern status of oral drug delivery systems including some of the recently evolved biotechnological/technical issues that are at a critical stage of seeking resolutions. The design engineering, and technologies that offer enhancements of the therapeutic opportunity with orally administered drugs were analyzed also.

6.1 Introduction to Oral Drug Administration

Oral drug delivery is the route of administering drugs that have been ingested and absorbed via the GI tract into systemic circulation. The process, however depends on pharmacokinetic principles where the drug has to dissolve in the GI fluids, permeate the intestinal lining, and eventually gain access to systemic circulation. This route has many influencing factors on how absorption and bioavailability may be influenced for orally administered drugs such as:
- ☐ Physicochemical Properties of Drugs: Solubility, Stability, and Molecular Size.
- ☐ All the above factors will affect the absorption of drugs.

- All factors: pH, enzyme activity, transit time, plays their role in determining both rate and extent of the drug absorption from GI Tract.
- First-Pass Metabolism: Drugs absorbed by the intestine go through the liver before they actually can reach systemic circulation, where they can be metabolized, hence reducing their effect.
- The primary goal of oral drug delivery systems is to maximize the amount of drug that ends up in the bloodstream in order to maximize efficacy while minimizing side effects.

6.2 Oral Drug Delivery Systems Advancement

Advances in materials science, engineering, and pharmacology have developed innovative oral delivery systems to improve drug stability, absorption, and release rates.

- **Modified-Release Formulations:** It controls the rate as well as location of drug release and provides therapeutic levels over extended periods with reduced frequency of dosing.

- **Extended-Release (ER) Systems**: ER tablets and capsules slowly and steadily release the drug for a prolonged effect in maintaining steady blood levels. It is most useful in managing chronic diseases like hypertension and diabetes, in which constant blood levels are of paramount importance.

Delayed-Release Systems: In these systems, the drug is released in a specific point of the GI tract. Delayed-release systems, such as enteric-coated tablets, avoid the release of the drug in the stomach, so acid-sensitive drugs are not degraded. Example: Some drugs, omeprazole, need DR systems to bypass the drug in the stomach and provide the delivery of the drug in the intestine.

- **Bioadhesive Systems:** Bioadhesive formulations adhere to the mucosal lining of the GI tract, increasing the contacting time of the drug with the absorption site and improving bioavailability. Mucoadhesive polymers in these systems help retain the drug in particular areas of the GI tract, thus enhancing the local concentration and absorption.

- **Nano-encapsulations and Nanoparticles:** Nano- and microparticle-based drug delivery systems protect drugs from enzymatic degradation and enhance absorption by increasing the surface area for interaction with the GI lining. Such formulations are useful for poorly soluble drugs since these drugs are dissolved more effectively in GI fluids.

- **Nanoparticles:** Nano-sized particles increase the absorption of drugs by crossing the cellular barriers. They also protect the drug from metabolic enzymes. Generally used for the drug delivery of anticancer drugs, which are very insoluble and have low bioavailability.

- **Microspheres and Microcapsules:** This system involves encapsulation of drugs within a polymer matrix for controlled or sustained release. Microspheres enable site-specific release from specific regions of the GI tract, thus enhancing the therapeutic impact of IBD diseases.

- **Prodrugs:** Prodrugs are pharmacologically inactive entities that become physiologically active upon metabolism in an organism. The chemical structure alterations of prodrugs enhance properties of solubility and stability of the drug molecule, thus improving its oral bioavailability. This strategy applies to drugs with poor GI absorption, such as some antiviral and anticancer agents, thus achieving therapeutic levels of drugs in the body.

- **Self-Emulsifying Drug Delivery Systems (SEDDS):** The formulation is based on lipid where emulsions form spontaneously in the GI tract thereby enhancing solubility and absorption. Bioavailability improves since the increase in drug solubibility increases, thus are more commonly used for lipophilic drugs that have the low absorption rate when the drug is orally ingested.

6.3 Biological and Physiological Challenges in Oral Delivery

With all that advancement, though, oral drug delivery still remains a hard nut for the body's natural defense mechanisms and GI physiology. Enzymatic Degradation: The breakdown of drugs in the GI tract by enzymes available, which include pepsin at the gastric level and proteases at the intestinal level. The latter mainly involves drugs derived from proteins or peptides. Variable pH: pH varies from acidic in the stomach to neutral to slightly alkaline in the intestines along the GI tract. It has an impact on drug stability and solubility. First-Pass Metabolism: Many drugs are degraded by the liver before they reach systemic circulation, which results in decreased levels of the active drug in the bloodstream. This process is known as first-pass metabolism. This limits drugs such as propranolol and nitroglycerin from achieving optimal bioavailability since extensive liver metabolism can degrade the drug. This would allow for limited absorption of large molecules, including hydrophilic peptides and proteins, not well absorbed into the intestinal lining; therefore, orally administered biologics, including insulin and some vaccines, would have limited efficacy.

6.4 Defeating Limitations through Innovated Technologies

Oral drug delivery has newer methods as well with still more scopes on the aspect of limitedness.

Permeation enhancers

Permeation enhancers agents which may momentarily open the tight junctions among intestinal cells. Examples are bile salts, fatty acids and surfactants. All these facilitate absorption for less permeable drugs.

Enzyme Inhibitors

Co-administration of enzyme inhibitors with specific drugs can slow down enzymatic degradation in the GI tract. This strategy is generally useful for protein and peptide drugs, which are subjected to significant enzymatic digestion.

Polymeric Coatings and Protective Layers
Advanced polymeric coatings protect drugs from stomach acid and digestive enzymes, improving stability and ensuring they reach the intestines intact. Polymers like Eudragit® are used in enteric coatings to shield drugs from acidic conditions, enabling controlled release at higher pH levels in the intestines.

Microneedle Capsules
One of the newly developed technologies in oral drug delivery is capsule-contained microneedles that can directly puncture the stomach wall or the intestinal lining and administer the drugs to the site where they otherwise would be destroyed in the GI tract due to their degradable properties.

6.5 Applications of Advanced Oral Drug Delivery Systems
Oral drug delivery innovations advance the applications scope of a great many medicines and bring treatment benefits of medical conditions in much improved ways.Extended and delayed release formulations are very effective in treating chronic diseases like diabetes, hypertension, and depression because they provide steady dosing for the patient and ensure compliance.

Cancer Therapy: Nanoformulations and prodrugs have allowed the oral delivery of chemotherapy agents that previously were administered intravenously, giving patients a more convenient treatment.

Viral and bacterial infections: Advanced formulations like SEDDS and bioadhesive systems can enhance the bioavailability of antiviral and antibiotic drugs to give better treatment for infections.

Pain Management: Modified-release opioid preparations, such as extended-release morphine, ensure long-term, sustained relief with minimal risks of side effects or addiction since it avoids peak dosing that is a hallmark of rapid-acting opioids. 10.6 Future Prospects in Oral Drug Delivery.

The future of oral drug delivery relates to the personalization of drug therapy, enhancing convenience of the patient, and treatments with improved efficacy.

Personalized Drug Delivery: Developing tailored oral formulations based on the genetics of patients for targeted drug delivery using recent developments in pharmacogenomics for optimizing dosage and minimizing adverse reactions.

Microbial Drug Delivery: Exploiting the human gastrointestinal microbiome as a drug delivery site can influence the microbiota and further enhance the efficacy of drugs administered orally.

Intelligent Oral Systems: Wearable devices and ingestible sensors can measure drug levels in real time, which allows for precise dosing and better treatment results.

Oral Delivery of Biologics: Scientists are working to develop the oral delivery systems of biologics such as insulin and vaccines so that patients do not have to inject. Oral drug delivery has been a part of modern medicine from the very beginning. Modern medicine continues to enhance and improve the bioavailability, stability, and efficacy of drugs administered orally.

Presently, advanced technologies are able to overcome the limitations that have been associated with the oral delivery systems and extend the therapeutic options in patients afflicted with chronic diseases or condition requiring precise and sustained medication. The future of oral drug delivery promises much more innovation toward making treatments more effective, convenient, and patient-friendly.

Chapter 7: Ocular Drug Delivery: Targeting Eye Diseases

Ocular drug delivery is one area of specialty that focuses the delivery of therapeutic agents to the eye-an organ that represents some unique challenges in the administration of drugs due to its complex anatomy and physiological barriers. Treatment of such eye diseases as glaucoma, age-related macular degeneration (AMD), diabetic retinopathy, and ocular infections demands highly specific drug delivery systems which can effectively penetrate the tissues of the eye and have minimal systemic side effects. It outlines the various delivery methods that entail ocular routes and includes every hurdle together with recent developments in the medical world.

7.1 Anatomy of the Eye and Barriers for Drug Delivery

To understand drug delivery in the eye, it is necessary to regard the anatomical and physiological features of the eye. Actually, the eye has several parts that are subdivided; each contains different barriers to permeation.

Cornea is the most peripheral covering of the eye and thus works as a primary protective layer in the process of topical drug delivery. It possesses five layers, such as epithelium, Bowman's layer, stroma, Descemet's membrane, and endothelium. Epithelium is hydrophobic at times that proves hard in achieving absorption through the site of hydrophilic drugs.

Conjunctiva: Thin membrane that coats the white part of the eye also known as the sclera, allows drug absorption, with high vascularity though, which causes drug clearance.

Aqueous Humor: This is the clear fluid that fills the anterior chamber of the eye. The aqueous humor is crucial in maintaining intraocular pressure and provides nutrients to intraocular structures.

Retina: The retina harbors the photoreceptor cells; an indispensable feature for vision. Drug delivery to the retina is peculiar because it restricts the passage of macromolecules and, consequently, potential drugs, due to the existence of the BRB.

All these obstacles bring into the delivery of a sufficiently working drug to the eye as great difficulty. So much so, it often cannot attain therapeutically active concentrations at the site through systemic or oral routes of administration.

7.2 Routes of Ocular Drug Delivery

Ocular drug delivery can broadly be classified into a number of routes, with some being advantageous and others less desirable:

Topical Delivery

The most common delivery technique of drugs into the eye is that of eye drops. In addition, eye drops contain often multiple drugs like anti-inflammatory agents, antibiotics or glaucoma drugs and their delivery is limited mostly because they are quickly sipped out from the eye and only about 5% of an instilled dose reaches the intraocular target.

Ointments and Gels: The formulations may prolong the contact time and absorption of the drug compared with conventional eye drops. Ointments have a longer duration of action but can obscure vision and create patient discomfort. Intraocular delivery

Intravitreal injections: Drugs are deposited intraocularly into the vitreous humor, giving this method the advantage of immediate action of the drug's very high concentration on both retina and vitreous; however, it means invasiveness, at possible risk of retinal detachment or hemorrhage.

Subconjunctival injections: Under this injection, a drug is administered below the conjunctiva that slowly drains into the eye. Subconjunctival injections are a bit less invasive compared to intravitreal but, certainly painful and lead to complications.

Systemic Delivery: Systemic administration, such as oral medication, can be used in certain conditions, though not the preferred route of ocular drug delivery. However, this case presents problems in attaining effective concentrations across the blood-ocular barrier. Sustained-release systems Implants and Inserts: These can also be used to administer the drugs over a period that may be long. So, the delivery of these drugs is not so frequent. Some examples are the biodegradable implants used for the delivery of agents with anti-VEGF to counter AMD over an extended period. Contact Lenses: Drug-eluting contact lenses are under development that can deliver therapeutic agents over time, providing a new method of ocular drug delivery and also their first purpose of vision correction.

7.3 Ocular Drug Delivery Challenges

Though there has been tremendous improvement in ocular drug delivery systems, challenges persist as follows:

Poor Penetration of Drugs: The multiple barriers formed by the cornea, conjunctiva, and BRB prevent efficient penetration of drugs into the ocular tissues.

Poor Retention Time: Frequent washout of drugs administered topically by tears and drainage results in poor bioavailability and frequent application.

Patient Compliance: The compliance of the patient will likely be compromised due to frequently administered dosing regimens; especially, this is in patients suffering from chronic conditions, such as glaucoma.

Side Effects: Systemic effects can be induced by ocular medications due to systemic drug absorption after topical administration. Drugs with potential systemic activity pose special considerations, especially the beta-blockers used to treat glaucoma patients.

7.4 Future Developments in Ocular Drug Delivery Technologies

Recent advancements in ocular drug delivery technologies are designed to overcome such issues and provide improved therapeutic results:

Nanotechnology

Nanoparticles, liposomes, and nanocarriers are being researched for ocular drug delivery as they are potential to enhance the solubility, stability, and permeation of drugs through ocular barriers. Polymeric nanoparticles, for example, can improve the bioavailability of hydrophilic drugs by enhancing their passage through the cornea.

Dissolving micro needles are considered the latest promising drug delivery through the ocular system. These very fine needles are introduced painlessly through the outer layers of the skin directly towards the target tissues, that are the retina. In most cases, it increases absorption in drugs without discomfort as well as other complications attributed to injections.

Sustained-Release Formulations

Some development related to formulation science has even led to sustained-release devices of hydrogels and implants that may ensure the uninterrupted release of the drug substance for long durations. One such example would be using hydrogels that undergo pH- or temperature-responsiveness drug release by which the drug release has been optimized and side effect lessened for more therapeutic outcome.

Smart Drug Delivery System

These systems are smart contact lenses, which have sensors measuring intraocular pressure or glucose levels and can release a medication on demand. This allows the possibility of personalized medicine during treatment for eye diseases, taking into consideration real-time physiological information about drug release.

7.5 Future Trends in Ocular Drug Delivery

As technology and research continue to expand and improve ocular drug delivery, there are multiple emerging trends and future directions:

Personalized Ocular Therapies: Advancements in genomics and proteomics can eventually personalize ocular therapy with regard to the individual's genetic profile and the specific ocular condition.

Therapeutic Combinations: Combination drug delivery is the simultaneous delivery of several therapeutic agents, which can potentially enhance the effectiveness of therapies targeted to complex eye diseases. The ocular drug delivery system that can deliver anti-inflammatory drugs and other growth factors together may present the combined effects of the therapies.

Ocular drug delivery systems may have a very critical role in regenerative medicine by utilizing stem cells or growth factors for the repair and regeneration of damaged ocular tissues.

Regulatory Issues: Regulatory concerns will be at a premium while new delivery systems are developed for safety, efficacy, and quality. The researchers, clinicians, and regulatory agencies must collaborate in order to move innovative therapies from bench to bedside.

Conclusion

Ocular drug delivery is one of the major research and development areas where the treatment of ocular diseases can be effectively handled, which may become much more important for patients' quality of life. Advances in drug delivery technologies will ensure ever-growing potential for even better, more patient-friendly, treatment options. Improvement of therapeutic outcomes will allow better ways for new drug developments in ophthalmology as well as improvement for more challenging, yet successful methods that are less complex through medical attention on ocular-specific drug delivery issues. Therefore, the future for the application of drug delivery system by drugs delivered into the eyes via nano scale technology and intelligent controlled devices with individualized, advanced patient care seems exciting in managing eye diseases more successfully.

Chapter: 8 Pulmonary Drug Delivery: Treating Respiratory Conditions

Pulmonary drug delivery is the administration of drugs directly to the lungs; it has become an indispensable part of respiratory disease treatment for patients with asthma, COPD, and cystic fibrosis. This method of drug delivery has numerous benefits: speed of absorption of drugs, significantly higher concentrations of drugs locally, and minimal systemic side effects. From being limited to just respiratory disorders, pulmonary delivery methods have now even emerged in systemic therapies such as diabetes and even certain cancers. The purpose of this chapter is to describe the science, development, and application of pulmonary drug delivery, focusing on its unparalleled role in modern medicine.

8.1. Anatomy and physiology of the respiratory tract as applied to drug delivery

Understanding the anatomy of the respiratory tract is important for designing optimal pulmonary drug delivery. The respiratory system comprises several different regions, each posing particular challenges and opportunities for drug absorption:

Upper Respiratory Tract: Includes the nasal cavity and pharynx; it first deals with most functions of filtering, warming, and humidifying inhaled air.

Conducting Airways: These include trachea, bronchi, and bronchioles, which guide air into the lungs. Drug particles will have to cross these conducting airways to reach the target areas of the lungs with maximum efficiency.

Alveolar Region: The alveoli are small air sacs in the lungs where gas exchange occurs. Due to their large surface area and thin epithelial barrier, the alveoli provide an ideal environment for drug absorption into the bloodstream.

The physiological characteristics of the respiratory system impact on designing pulmonary drug delivery systems and their effectiveness. Effective delivery overcomes the natural barriers while allowing drugs to reach the site desired in sufficient concentrations.

8.2 Pulmonary drug delivery and its advantages

Pulmonary drug delivery provides unique benefits that set apart the pulmonary route from others in treating respiratory conditions and beyond:

Direct delivery to the target site: In respiratory diseases, direct delivery of drugs to the lungs increases local concentrations and maximizes efficacy with reduced dose.

Quickly acting: The large surface area and rich blood supply ensure quick absorption through the lungs, so drugs can act in speedy fashion. This feature is particularly useful in such acute conditions as asthma attacks.

Lowered Systemic Side Effects: Direct targeting of the lung reduces systemic exposure hence lowers the incidence of systemic side effects of oral or intravenous drugs.

Potential for Systemic Delivery: A drug delivered to the alveolar region is capable of systemic absorption and thus treatment of systemic diseases. For example, insulin has been explored for pulmonary delivery for systemic control of diabetes.

8.3. Types of Pulmonary drug delivery systems:Pulmonary drug delivery involves many different devices, each with a different mechanism of application:

Metered dose inhalers: The metered dose inhaler is perhaps the most commonly used device for lung-delivered drugs. The patient inhales a propellant that aerosolizes a fixed dose of medication and then delivers it into the lungs. MDIs are very portable and convenient when used with short- and long-acting bronchodilators.

Dry Powder Inhalers: DPIs deliver powdered drugs in two ways without propellants. However, DPIs use a different delivery mechanism where inhaled powder is deposited into the lungs subsequently. DPIs are more often selected for preparations whose stability is maintained in dry form and which can be used for maintenance therapy of chronic respiratory diseases. Nebulizers: A nebulizer changes liquid medication to an aerosol mist for breathing by patients. Nebulizers are less portable than a device, such as an inhaler, but do deliver much more and are often suggested in severe exacerbations or situations.

Soft Mist Inhalers: In SMIs, the pharmaceutical agent is delivered as a fine mist of droplets thus easily taken in. SMIs do not contain propellants. Increased penetration through the lungs enhances the efficiency of drug delivery since the release of the mist is slower. The specific benefits of each system also have the specific limitations that would govern the selection process based on patient preference, type of drug, and the disease.

8.4. Pulmonary Formulations of Drugs

It is important since the drug may considerably influence the site of location and how well the formulation will be absorbed depending on the characteristics of the particles. The factors to include are:

Particle Size: Particle size determines how deep into the lungs the drug may penetrate. Particles that range from 1 to 5 micrometers are ideal for reaching the lower airways and alveoli, whereas bigger particles tend to deposit in the upper airways.

Stability and Solubility: Drugs need to be stable and sufficiently soluble to maintain their action within the respiratory tract. Lipophilic drugs need to be carried or emulsified to increase their solubility.

Aerosolization Properties: The aerosol formability is very crucial for the drugs used in inhalers and nebulizers. The aerosolization performance of these drugs can be enhanced by incorporating additives or excipients into the formulation.

The next advancement was in controlled release, which led to formulating the idea that drugs can act over an extended period, thereby reducing the administration frequency and improving patient compliance.

8.5. Pulmonary Drug Delivery Applications

The primary application for pulmonary drug delivery remains respiratory diseases, although systemic conditions have been approached and researched recently.

Pulmonary treatment remains the core of asthma and COPD management. Here, bronchodilators, corticosteroids, or combination therapy come in the form of an inhalation device for easy rapid relief and long-term control.

Aerosol antibiotics: Like tobramycin, are administered to cystic fibrosis patients with chronic infections, whereas aerosol mucolytic drugs dissolve the thickened mucus that can be coughed or suctioned out of the lungs.

Pulmonary Hypertension: Here, prostacyclins are administered through inhalation that can dilate blood vessels in the lungs and thus reduce pulmonary blood pressure to alleviate symptoms of pulmonary hypertension.

Diabetes: Insulin administered through the lungs is promising for managing the glucose levels in blood in patients suffering from diabetes. It is not an invasive process since it injects insulin into the bloodstream.

Vaccines and Gene Therapy: Inhaled vaccines are under development as a means to promote immunity against such respiratory pathogens as influenza or SARS-CoV-2 through direct targeting at the site of the lungs. In addition, inhaled gene therapies are being studied in the management of genetic pulmonary diseases.

8.6. Pulmonary Drug Delivery Issues

Despite the potential benefits of pulmonary drug delivery, there are some inherent challenges preventing its extensive use:

Maintain unconsistency in the dose: Since pulmonary circulation is rather variable, depending on the different variations in breathing patterns of the individual, lung capacity, and pathological state, it becomes troublesome to maintain consistency in the dose.

Patient Technique and Compliance: Inadequate delivery from the drug is often the result of poor inhaler technique. Most patients misuse an inhaler, so patient education and device innovation are required to improve patient compliance.

Formulation stability: Many of the drugs are sensitive to ambient conditions or may degrade during transit across the lung, and consequently, their efficiency becomes limited. This is a greatly studied area in stabilization of such formulations.

Local respiratory side effects : While it may reduce systemic side effects from pulmonary delivery, local respiratory side effects like throat irritation, coughing, or bronchospasm could still occur, especially from an inhaled corticosteroid or a strong bronchodilator.

8.7. Pulmonary drug delivery: Future directions

Research in pulmonary drug delivery continues to evolve, with several promising directions for future advancements:

Nanoparticles and Liposome-Based Inhalation Therapies: Nanoparticles and liposomes can encapsulate drugs and protect them from degradation and enhance the drugs' ability to reach targeted lung regions. Liposome-based formulations have already shown success in treating certain lung infections.

Smarter inhalers: Smarter inhalers have a sensor and connective properties, which allow for in-real-time monitoring of patient use of inhalers; it is crucial for better management of chronic conditions by patients. They can monitor patterns, remind patients, and provide reports that help healthcare providers to better adhere to treatment leading to improved outcomes.

Personalized medicine: Personalized medicine will improve the pulmonary drug delivery system. The ability to be tailored according to the patients' genetics, lung functions, and disease characteristics can progress a more effective treatment with lower side effects.

Pulmonary delivery of RNA and gene-based therapies: Stable, inhalable RNA and DNA therapeutic systems have a bright future in treating genetic lung diseases, such as cystic fibrosis. Direct delivery of gene-editing tools, like CRISPR, to the lung may unlock completely new paradigms of therapy for correction of genetic defects at their source.

Inhaled vaccines: There is renewed interest in inhaled vaccines to prime mucosal immunity within the lung itself where the respiratory pathogens often enter, with all the devastation caused by the COVID-19 pandemic. Inhaled vaccines may also provide more robust and longer-lasting immunity for the immunized subjects than injectable vaccines for respiratory viruses.

Conclusion: Pulmonary drug delivery has changed the face of managing respiratory diseases using direct, local administration with rapid onset of action and minimal systemic side effects. New formulations and devices have been emerging and driving the field into more challenging applications beyond just respiratory diseases; into systemic conditions, to genetic therapies, and ultimately to vaccines. Though there exist problems such as formulation stability and compliance by the patient, the future of pulmonary drug delivery sounds promising, and advancement in technology has developed this route of administration even more refined and personalized.

Chapter 9 Injectable Drug Delivery Systems: Improving Patient Compliance

Injectable drug delivery systems might well be the most common form of therapeutic delivery, with direct access into the bloodstream, allowing for fast, accurate drug delivery. Though injectable are often thought of in terms of needles and syringes, injectable drug delivery encompasses a very wide range of devices and approaches aimed at improving the patient experience and increasing compliance. This chapter explores the main types of injectable systems, how they work, advantages and limitations, and some recent developments toward minimizing pain, convenience, and improved treatment outcome for the patient.

9.1 Introduction to Injectable Drug Delivery Systems

It is defined as drug delivery by administering drugs directly into the body through injection routes. The most common types involve subcutaneous under the skin, intramuscular in the muscle, intravenous into the vein, and intradermal into the skin injection methods. Such modes are particularly beneficial when the medication would be degraded by the gastrointestinal tract, cannot be absorbed effectively, or needs to produce its effect rapidly. Despite the advantages, injectable systems have been characterized by pain, inconvenience, and the psychological dislike that many patients have for needles. These have motivated advanced injection devices and formulations that increase compliance in patients and facilitate self-administration.

9.2 Types of Injectable Drug Delivery Systems

Conventional Syringes and Needles

The most common injectable system used is the conventional syringe, from vaccinations to insulin. While effective, these systems can sometimes be painful, and patients with conditions requiring daily injection courses, such as diabetes or hormone replacement therapies, may find adhering to these a trial.

Prefilled Syringes and Autoinjectors

Prefilled syringes have a ready-to-use advantage in minimizing the error associated with dosing and reducing preparation time, thus beneficial to the patient as well as the health care provider. An autoinjector is a device that enables a patient to self-administer a dose precisely with just the touch of a button. The autoinjectors are highly popular in the biologics and the treatments of chronic diseases, like rheumatoid arthritis, which will help the patient administer treatment without much hassle.

Pen Injectors

Pen injectors are portable and ambulatory devices mainly used by patients with conditions requiring hormone therapy, such as for insulin. They are dose flexible, have a minimum usage requirement, and may be set for single or multiple dosing. The ergonomic design of pen injectors, and its simplified dosage adjustments, promote patient compliance even with such an ordeal for diabetes patients.

Needle-Free Injectors

Needles are not used in needle-free injectors. It employs high-pressure air or liquid to inject the drug through the skin without a needle. This system is aimed to remove anxiety and discomfort related to needles, hence increasing the patient compliance. Though this system was initially available for a few types of vaccines and insulin, with modernization of the needle-free technology, it is applied in a wider context.

Implantable and Depot Injectable Systems

Implantable devices and long-acting injectable systems, commonly known as depot injectables, release medication slowly for extended periods. They suit chronic conditions like schizophrenia, which patients may find it challenging to adhere to their daily or weekly medication regimes. Depot injections reduce dosing frequency to monthly or quarterly intervals, thus improving compliance in long-term treatments.

9.3 Key Routes of Injection

Every injection route has its specific roles in drug delivery. It affects the drug's effectiveness, speed of action, and comfort to the patient based on the chosen route.

Intravenous (IV) Injection:

In this route, the medicine is injected directly into the blood where it is needed urgently and hastens its action. IV injections are common in emergency circumstances, chemotherapy, and any other situation that requires prompt results.

Intramuscular Injection:
Depot of medicines injected into muscles are absorbed into the blood quite rapidly, used for vaccines and a few antibiotics. Though far more painful, they are useful for drugs where a rate is required that is slower than IV but more rapid than subcutaneous.

Subcutaneous (SC) Injection:
Subcutaneous injections administer drug into the tissue beneath your skin for slow, gradual absorption. SC injections are preferred in treatments wherein the drugs are released gradually, like in managing diabetes with injectable insulin and some vaccinations. It's less painful and more favored for administration on one's self.

Intradermal (ID) Injection:
Intradermal injections administer drugs in the outer layers of skin and are used for diagnostics and allergy testing. Due to limited absorption, ID injections are not typically used for therapeutic drugs but have been particularly helpful in vaccine formulation and testing.

9.4 Advantages of Injectable Drug Delivery Systems
Injectable systems offer an unique set of advantages for drugs that require rapid onset or have poor oral bioavailability:

Rapid Absorption:

Injections allow for quick uptake of drugs into the blood, which can help establish a rapid therapeutic effect. In emergency medicine, speed can literally be a lifesaver.

No Gastrointestinal First-Pass Effect:
Injectable routes bypass the gastrointestinal tract and therefore avoid problems associated with enzymatic degradation of drugs; thus some drugs that might exhibit poor bioavailability, such as proteins and peptides, would never reach any systemic circulation if administered orally.

Sustained and Targeted Release:
The injectable systems, especially depot injections and implantable devices, provide the slowly released drug for a longer period of time, which reduces the dosing frequency. This concept of sustained release is particularly useful in treating chronically debilitating diseases like schizophrenia, where constant drug concentration becomes essential for some drugs for effectiveness.

9.5 Challenges and Limitations of Injectable Systems

Injectable drug delivery systems have many advantages, but there are also some limitations that may discourage patients from using them.

Pain and Discomfort:
Pain and discomfort are still the main barriers to patient compliance because of fear of needles and pain caused by injections, particularly in therapies that need frequent injections.

Risk of Infection and Injury:
Misuse injection technique can lead to infections or tissue damage from the site of injection. In addition to this, self-injecting users are liable to be "stuck with the needle", assuming proper disposal has not been utilized.

Training and Access: Many injectable devices require training which may make self-injection procedure difficult. Also, the accessibility of a trained healthcare professional may not be easy and may be available to only those users who stay in the low resource environment making self-administered scheduled injections infeasible.

9.6 Injectable Drug Delivery Innovations
The recent advances made in injectable systems are essentially to reduce pain, cut down the dosing frequencies, and make self- administration easier.

Micro-Needle Patches
These patches contain micro needles that only penetrate the epidermis for pain free drug delivery. Micro -needle patches were originally developed to deliver vaccines but are now being applied to chronic conditions.

Self-Healing Hydrogels:
Researchers are working on injectable hydrogels that form a stable depot at the injection site and slowly release the drug. Such hydrogels can be used for localized treatments in diseases such as cancer and tissue regeneration.

Long-Acting Injectable (LAI) Formulations:
LAIs are long-acting formulations that deliver drugs over weeks or even months, making it more convenient and adherent. LAIs are being used in HIV, schizophrenia, and hormone replacement therapies to avoid frequent dosing.

Smart Injectors:
Digital Integration Smart injectors are combined with digital technology and can report on patient adherence, dose, and even physiological markers that can be sent back to health care providers. Such real-time monitoring is highly important in disease conditions that require strict adherence, such as multiple sclerosis or cardiovascular diseases.

9.7 Case Studies: Injectable Systems in Practice

Ozempic (Semaglutide): It is a subcutaneous injection for Type 2 diabetes and administered once a week. It has proven to be so effective in achieving sugar control among patients. Its dosing requirement only once a week makes it more convenient for the patient than daily injections.

Prolia (Denosumab): Given subcutaneously every six months in osteoporosis treatment, Prolia makes dosing much easier; compliance is high because the dosing administrations are less frequent, so the risks for missed treatments are lower.

Abilify Maintena: Abilify Maintena is administered monthly as an extended-release intramuscular injection for the treatment of schizophrenia. Long-acting antipsychotic injectables such as Abilify Maintena are beneficial for those who cannot adhere to daily oral dosing, as it ensures the constant delivery of therapeutic benefits and minimizes the likelihood of relapse.

9.8 Future Directions in Injectable Drug Delivery

Injectable drug delivery continues to advance with the emphasis being placed on making systems more user-friendly for patients.

Wearable injectors, or on-body delivery systems, are a type of delivery system that adheres to the skin and delivers medication over a prolonged period. They are most useful for high-volume drugs that cannot be delivered in one injection and are typically used in the treatment of cancer and autoimmune conditions.

Bio-Inspired Injection Devices: From nature to man, these devices try to emulate the painless sting of some insects. Thus, a fundamental approach may benefit injection techniques with truly painless needles and raises the compliance from needle-phobic patients.

Personalized and 3D-Printed Injectables: Advances in 3D printing will allow for fully customized, patient-specific injectable devices. Thus, personalized injectables will be developed and tailored to deliver best dosages that are based on each individual's metabolic and therapeutic needs.

Dual and Multi-Drug Delivery Systems: Future injectable systems will perhaps be devised to deliver multiple drugs together. This approach is deemed a favorable strategy in cancer treatment because the combination treatment proves often to be better than any single treatment.

Chapter 10 Controlled-Release Systems: Improving Therapeutic Outcomes

The first revolution in modern medicine, controlled-release drug delivery systems release drugs at predetermined and controlled rates over a long period. In this manner, controlled-release delivery systems overcome the inadequacies of conventional drug administration by reducing the demand for multiple doses within short intervals, decrease unwanted side effects at target sites, and maintain constant levels of drugs in the bloodstream. Controlled-release drug delivery systems hold vast applications in chronic disease treatments, pain management, cancer therapy, etc. This chapter addresses the science behind controlled-release systems, types of systems used, and an influence exerted on therapeutic outcomes.

10.1. Overview of Controlled-Release Systems

Controlled-release systems are designed to enhance the drug's delivery and absorption within the body. These systems, by controlling the release rate, ensure a consistent level of the drug at therapeutic levels and thus do not produce peaks and troughs associated with immediate-release formulations. Advantages include increased efficacy, enhanced compliance among patients, less frequent dosing, and, in most cases, decreased side effects. The key objectives of controlled-release systems include

Optimal Therapeutic Levels: A steady level of the drug in the bloodstream is necessary for an optimal treatment where their levels may fluctuate and compromise the efficacy of the drug or cause adverse effects.

Infrequent Dosing: This will enhance compliance on the part of the patients with chronic disorders where long-term maintenance therapy is required.

Side Effect Minimization: Controlled release can also prevent the initial "burst" of drug concentration found in immediate-release systems that results in undesirable side effects.

10.2. Classifications of Controlled-Release Systems

Controlled release may be achieved through mechanisms and system designs. Types most commonly used are classified into matrix systems, reservoir systems, osmotic systems, and biodegradable systems each having some inherent advantage for specific therapeutic use.

Matrix Systems: Here, the drug is dispersed uniformly in a polymer matrix. The drug diffuses through the matrix material at a slow rate so that a gradual release of the drug can take place over a period of time. Matrix systems are often used in oral tablets, transdermal patches, and implantable devices. The rate of release can be varied by altering the properties of the matrix material, for example, porosity and type of polymer.

In reservoir systems: The central core of the drug is enclosed by a membrane. This membrane controls and regulates the release of drug. By adjusting the release rate of drugs through the membrane, which can be modified either by making the membrane thicker or changing its composition, reservoir systems find wide application in the design of transdermal patches and implantable devices. Drugs are released steadily and over long periods of days, weeks, or even months.

Osmotic Systems: These delivery systems rely on osmosis to deliver a drug. In these devices, the process of osmosis creates water entry into the device via a semipermeable membrane. This is known to create pressure that consequently expels the drug via a small orifice. In this system, the drug delivery rate is very predictable and does not depend upon environment-related pH or movement conditions; hence, it goes perfectly well with oral tablets, which have to deposit the exact calculated dosages within the gastrointestinal tract.

Biodegradable Systems: Biodegradable controlled-release systems are formulated using materials that biodegrade in vivo, with the rate of degradation governed by the intended application. Materials commonly used include PLGA. As the formulation degrades, drug delivery is achieved. Biodegradable systems are mainly utilized with implantable devices, as well as in oncology to produce localized, sustained-release. The biodegradable systems eliminate the need for surgical device removal once the drug supply is depleted.

10.3. Mechanism of Drug Release in Controlled-Release Systems

The release mechanisms in controlled-release systems may vary with material composition, device design, and the intended application. Some of the primary release mechanisms include:

Diffusion-Controlled Release: In diffusion-controlled systems, a drug is released as it diffuses through a polymer barrier. Release can be either in matrix or reservoir systems as the drug can diffuse through the matrix material or the reservoir membrane. The rate of diffusion can also be modified by changing the properties of the polymer.

Dissolution-Controlled Release: In dissolution-controlled systems, the dissolution rate of a drug or of a coating material determines the rate of release. For instance, tablets with a slow outer layer that dissolves can gradually dissolve and in the process release the drug to the body to control exposure rates.

Osmosis-Controlled Release: Water diffuses in through a semipermeable membrane in osmotic systems and puts pressure on the drug within through the orifice. This system provides an extremely reliable, steady release rate that does not respond to external conditions.

Erosion-Controlled Release: For this class of biodegradable system, the rate of release is essentially proportional to erosion or material degradation. This makes it a particularly useful technology for implantable devices where drug delivery is required over weeks or even months at a gradual, steady rate.

10.4 Applications of Controlled-Release Systems

Controlled release of systems has wide applications across various medical disciplines because of its ability to enhance drug efficacy and improve the quality of life for patients.

Most chronic diseases for example diabetes, hypertension, and asthma, require steady drug levels that will be managed over an extensive period of time. Control-released medication delivery preserves the therapeutic ranges while the rate of the dosing can be brought down to minimal. Examples include: For example, when using the oral form called Metformin XR on type 2 diabetes drugs, maintains normal blood sugar levels for even fewer infrequent dosages during the course of the day.

Pain Management: Chronic pain management requires controlled-release formulations in which steady drug levels provide relief without the peaks and troughs associated with immediate-release medications. Extended-release formulations of opioids like oxycodone and morphine help to provide long-lasting relief from pain and decrease the need for frequent dosing.

Oncology: A controlled release is used in delivering chemotherapeutic agents directly to a tumor site, preventing healthy tissues from exposure to the chemotherapeutic agent and reducing systemic side effects. Implantable drug delivery devices with controlled release capabilities can provide sustained local drug release over time and are especially useful for sites that are hard to access, such as tumors located behind the eye or sometimes within the brain.

Neurological Diseases: Drugs in controlled-release are useful in diseases like Parkinson's and epilepsy, where a stable drug level could prevent the fluctuation that leads to induction of symptoms. Examples of Levodopa-extended formulations help Parkinson's patients to have stability in motor functions which can be sustained for an extended period of time.

Stable levels of drugs can be delivered with injectable controlled-release systems, implants, or patches to provide steady drug concentration, which is important in controlling chronic infections like HIV and tuberculosis. For example, long-acting antiretrovirals injections prevent HIV patients from experiencing drug re-bound, hence increasing patient compliance with fewer dosages. Though controlled-release systems bring many benefits, it has its challenges as well. Here are some benefits and potential pitfalls.

Benefits:
Easy Adherence for Patients with Chronic Disease: Controlled release can limit dosing time; thereby enhancing patient adherence to prescribed regimens

Fewer Side Effects: Consistent therapeutic levels suppress the burst in drug exposure during an initial release by an immediate release formulation to prevent or decrease side effects

Effective Treatments: Patients achieve more desirable and effective therapy by obtaining more consistent and prolonged exposure to therapeutic doses

10.5 Limitations:

Complex Manufacturing: Controlled-release systems are often more expensive as they require complex manufacturing and engineering processes.

Risk of Dose Dumping: Dose dumping is a high risk when a controlled release system fails or is tampered with. Dose dumping refers to the unintended and rapid release of the drug, which can be unsafe.

Limited Applicability to Some Drugs: Not all drugs can be formulated into controlled-release systems. Drugs with narrow therapeutic windows, rapid metabolism, or instability in various pH conditions are not suitable for controlled-release systems.

10.6. Future Developments in Controlled-Release Systems
Current research and technological advancements are continually improving the possibility of controlled-release systems. These include:

Smart Polymers: Responsive or smart polymers can release drugs according to specific stimuli, either temperature, pH, or enzymes. These polymers made drug release on demand become excellent for precision medicine application.

Nanotechnology Incorporation: Nanoscale control-release systems can be addressed at particular tissues or cell layers. Thus, better accuracy and efficacy in terms of drug delivery can result from such nanoscale systems. Nanoparticles are being developed so as to cross the blood-brain barrier. Thus new pathways in the treatment process for neurological diseases will start to emerge.

Wearable devices: Its use controlled-release technology are monitored and adjusted in real-time based on patient conditions. For example, insulin pumps are now designed with feedback systems that alter dosing based on glucose levels.

The Future of Controlled-Release Systems: Tailoring Devices and Formulations to Individual Patient Needs. The future of controlled-release systems lies in tailoring devices and formulations to individual patient needs. Personalized controlled-release systems could adjust drug delivery rates based on patient metabolism, age, weight, and other factors to optimize therapeutic outcomes.

Conclusion:
This chapter presents how controlled-release systems improved therapeutic outcomes for a vast variety of medical

conditions. These systems basically enhance the stability of a drug, decrease side effects, and ensure constant levels of a drug. At every step of research advancement, controlled-release systems can be advanced to be that much more precise, sensitive, and patient-specific for maximum treatment benefit. After this chapter shall be discussion on gene therapy and viral vectors as breakthroughs in drug delivery-what exactly is done with those emerging genetic therapies.

Chapter 11 Polymers In Drug Delivery: Enhancing Drug Efficacy And Stability

Nowadays, with extensive research on polymers as one of the versatile and necessary materials in drug delivery systems, these can enhance stability, control the release rate of the drug, bioavailability, and compliance. Polymers can also be designed into different structures that include nanoparticles, hydrogels, and matrix systems with highly sensitive conditions to adjust the timing and location as well as quantity of the drug release. This chapter discusses the types of polymers used in drug delivery, their functions, applications, and the latest advancements that demonstrate their role in transforming medical treatments, particularly in chronic and complex conditions.

11. Overview of Polymers in Drug Delivery

The role of polymers in drug delivery systems is multifaceted and goes beyond simple encapsulation of drugs. Their structures can be engineered to enhance the therapeutic effects of drugs while reducing their potential side effects, making them a basis for new approaches in drug design and patient care. Key benefits include:

Encapsulation of Drugs: The encapsulation of drugs within polymers protects them from enzymatic or environmental degradation, improving the stability and efficacy of drugs, particularly biologics or drugs that are pH or temperature sensitive.

Controlled Release: It is possible to engineer polymers so that the composition and structure are tailored such that they deliver drugs at specific times; hence, they are well suited for chronic diseases where continuous dosing is required.

Targeted Delivery: If attached with targeting ligands, drugs can be directly delivered to specific tissues or cells, such as cancer cells, resulting in reduced systemic exposure and further adverse effects.

Since polymers are versatile material, they are designed into various applications that include polymeric nanoparticles, hydrogels, degradable implants, and matrix systems, all of which have different beneficial properties.

11.2. Forms of Polymers used for drug delivery

Polymers that are used for drug delivery fall into the general categories of natural, synthetic, and semi-synthetic. Each type possesses unique characteristics suited to certain applications.

Natural Polymers: The most common source of naturally occurring polymers is biological entities, and natural polymers are biocompatible along with being biodegradable. Some examples of common natural polymers include: Chitosan Alginate Hyaluronic Acid Gelatin In the previous discussion, it has been outlined that natural polymers will find a wider application within the field of wound healing applications, tissue engineering applications, or even drug delivery systems needing the least possible toxicity in terms of interaction with natural substances. Chitosan-based nanoparticles are used especially for nasal as well as transdermal drug delivery systems because of their mucoadhesive property.

Synthetic Polymers: PLGA, PEG, and PCL are used synthetic polymers. They show tailor-made capabilities along with controlled degradation rates. Most of the controlled release systems as well as drug targeting, specifically in cancer therapy, need very specific targeting along with controlled release.

Semi-Synthetic Polymers: Semi-synthetic polymers, cellulose derivatives, for example, hydroxypropyl methylcellulose or HPMC, enhance drug solubility and stability and have become useful in the preparation of oral drug delivery formulations and also improved bioavailability.

11.3. Polymeric Nanoparticles in Drug Delivery

Polymeric nanoparticles, mostly less than 200 nanometers in diameter, have emerged as an efficient delivery vehicle for drugs, where controlled release and targeted delivery are possible while providing drugs with protection from degradation.

Biodegradability and Biocompatibility: Most of the polymeric nanoparticles are biodegradable. They break down to innocuous products, which means nontoxic products that degrade in the body, including PLGA. This results in degradation products, lactic and glycolic acids, which are naturally metabolized in the body and are nontoxic and safe for prolonged usage in sustained release therapy.

High Encapsulation Efficiency. Polymeric nanoparticles provide an encapsulation capacity, where there is a higher amount of more drugs that will go to the target. A good efficiency will ensure fewer and reduced side effects for a better output in a therapy.

Controlled release of drugs: The rate of drug release from polymeric nanospheres could be controlled by the molecular weight or composition of the polymer. This would provide either immediate or sustained release, to be matched according to the needs of the patient.

11.4. Hydrogels: Elastic Polymer-Based Delivery Systems

Hydrogels are cross-linked, hydrophilic polymer networks that contain large volumes of water or biological fluids. High water content and a soft structure give hydrogels biocompatibility and enable them to adapt to the range of applications from wound care to the localized drug delivery.

Responsive Hydrogels: These hydrogels are also called "smart" hydrogels. These polymers deliver the drugs in an environment-sensitive manner due to the response of temperature, pH variations, or light. For example, pH-sensitive hydrogels deliver their payload at acidic values, similar to those of tumor cells or inflamed tissues.

Injectable Hydrogels: Liquid at room temperature, which becomes a solid upon being injected in the body; thus they can be designed for minimal-invasive therapies such as local drug delivery in cancer treatment or the healing of surgical wounds as therapeutic agents can be released from them right at the place of the therapy.

Sustained Drug Release: Hydrogels can be used to release drugs for a long time. It is very useful in chronic conditions that require steady levels of therapy, such as diabetes, where insulin-loaded hydrogels provide steady hormone release.

11.5. Biodegradable Implants and Polymer Matrices

Such devices are useful for chronic drug application in the management of pain, hormone replacement therapy, and other types of tumors that require implants for long time periods. The polymer matrix has the advantage of its design to be biodegradable in order to ensure targeted delivery of drugs in this case.

Polymeric Implants: The drugs slowly get released from the polymer as it degrades. PLGA implants are used for delivering chemotherapy drugs to the tumor site itself to deliver targeted therapy with minimum side effects. Since the polymer degrades with time, surgical removal is not necessary after treatment.

Matrix Systems: The drug is dispersed in a polymer matrix system that gradually diffuses into the scaffold, and this is a sustained-release system. These systems are commonly used in wound care applications whereby, the polymer matrix facilitates an even release of the antibiotic or anti-inflammatory to accelerate healing.

11.6. Application of Polymers in Drug Delivery

The versatility of polymers has led to their use in various medical fields where they improve the outcome of treatment and minimize side effects.

Chemotherapy: Polymeric nanoparticles are used in chemotherapy. They are used for targeted delivery of drugs directly to the tumor cells, thereby minimizing the damage to healthy tissues. For example, PLGA nanoparticles are used for the encapsulation of drugs such as paclitaxel and doxorubicin. These nanoparticles enable targeted treatment with reduced toxicity.

Use for diabetes management: Hydrogels and other polymeric systems are under study for a controlled delivery of insulin for reducing the injection frequency by diabetic patients, and there is a responsive, controlled release system to improve the glucose control.

Ocular drug delivery: Polymers are used in eye drop, implants, and lenses to provide the gradual delivery of drugs; this might be helpful for glaucoma patients because these patients will maintain a steady pressure inside their eyes.

Vaccine Delivery: polymeric nanoparticles demonstrated the ability to enhance the efficiency of a vaccine by directly providing antigens to cells of the immune system. Vaccine delivery with lipid-based formulation systems could be a future alternative in those cases in view of COVID-19 and disease similar to that.

Neurological Disorders: certain categories of polymers are being used as crossing Blood-Brain Barriers vehicles to deliver drugs in diseases related to cognitive disorders, which includes Alzheimer's/Parkinson's. A treatment by drug delivery using anti-inflammatory peptides with PEGylated nanoparticles can provide better therapy than with the previously applied methods in the central nervous system.

11.7. Case Studies: Polymers in Clinical Practice

Lupron Depot® (PLGA Microspheres): This drug delivery system offers a hormone therapy medication, leuprolide acetate for several months through PLGA microspheres that provide a sustained release of the drug. A drug whose application in prostate cancer has been popular and also found useful in the treatment of endometriosis, Lupron Depot is one of the prime examples of polymers used to achieve compliance through minimum dosing.

Zoladex®: Biodegradable Implant (Zoladex): This has an implant that is embedded with goserelin for cancer treatment of the prostate and breasts. Over time, these implants continuously release drugs thereby providing steady treatment without frequent efforts from a patient.)

Ozurdex® (Intravitreal Implant): A PLGA-based implant for Ozurdex, which uses dexamethasone to be intravitreal. Ozurdex therefore helps treat conditions such as macular edema and uveitis using a fixed dose of corticosteroid drugs intravitrealy without recurring eye injection.

11.8. Future of Polymers in Drug Delivery

Polymers are developed and advanced with new scientific findings as well as new technologies that will allow for more efficient, individualized treatments.

Personalized Polymer Systems: Future developments in the field might focus on tailoring systems patient-by-patient individually constructed from polymers. Strikingly, specific manipulation of polymer composition and rates of degradation may be able to direct release profiles of drugs incorporated within to an end, creating truly personalized care.

Self-healing polymers : The ability of self-healing means that they can potentially heal minor damage, and so long-lasting implants or hydrogels with consistent drug delivery would be possible in such a complex environment as the digestive system.

Bio-inspired and biomimetic polymers: Even more dramatic improvements in compatibility and efficacy for applications as complex as blood-brain barrier penetration can be realized if natural structures are mimicked by these polymers.

Multitasking polymers: Polymers are engineered to serve various functions not only for delivery of drugs but also the monitoring of biological conditions and response to stimuli, capable of adjusting in terms of the time course in treatment and moving towards personalized therapy.

Chapter 12- Biodegradable Systems: The Future Of Sustainable Drug Delivery

Biodegradable drug delivery systems form the substrates of environment-friendly and patient-friendly therapies in the process of development. They naturally reduce long-time impacts, diminish the necessity of removal surgeries, and deliver drugs to desired sites with high precision and efficacy. This chapter reviews the various types of biodegradable systems, mechanisms, medical field applications, and innovation in moving forward with the technology.

12.1 Introduction to Biodegradable Systems for Drug Delivery

The systems are designed to have an intended purpose for a time, then degrade into non-toxic byproducts that can be naturally removed from the body. These systems find most of their applications in chronic disease management, post-surgical treatments, and localized drug delivery, wherein a prolonged therapeutic presence would be beneficial. Biodegradable systems come in all shapes and sizes, with forms including microspheres, nanoparticles, implants, and hydrogels, all geared for specific delivery needs.

Important Benefits: Less Surgical Intervention Required: Because biodegradable systems are self-dissolving, no surgical intervention will be needed to remove these, which means less surgery for patients and reduced costs on health care.

Release of Drug: Most biodegradable systems have a drug release over an extended period with levels that remain at therapeutically acceptable concentrations

Minimizing Impact to Environment: Biodegradable materials decompose with less leaving residues that would contribute to the harm of the environment

12.2 Types of Biodegradable System
Various biodegradable systems possess characteristic properties and uses: some of the most important types that have obtained a great deal of interest in recent studies are listed below.

12.2.1. Biodegradable Polymers
- **Poly(lactic-co-glycolic acid) (PLGA):** PLGA is one of the most widely used biodegradable polymers. It has many applications in drug delivery, including the preparation of microspheres and nanoparticles. It degrades into lactic and glycolic acids, which are naturally metabolized within the body.
- **Polylactic Acid (PLA):** PLA is widely used, owing to its high tensile strength and biocompatibility. Applications include sutures, implants, and drug delivery formulations, that degrade slowly.
- **Polycaprolactone (PCL):** PCL degrades slowly hence it is used in prolonged release applications like an orthopedic implant, and for chronic disease management.

12.2.2. Hydrogels

- **Natural Biodegradable Hydrogels:** Obtained from natural biopolymers, such as hydrogels based on chitosan, alginate, and collagen, Natural hydrogels maintain moisture within the wound, ensuring wound healing and tissue formation take place.

- **Synthetic Biodegradable Hydrogels:** Synthetic biodegradable hydrogels manufactured through PEG, for instance, are specifically designed with inherent degradability in situations involving changes in temperature or a sudden shift in pH

12.2.3. Biodegradable Nanoparticles and Microspheres

- **PLGA or PLA-based nanoparticles and microspheres**: These can encapsulate drugs ranging from small molecules to large proteins. This indicates that the drug delivery could be targeted and controlled. These are used in cancer treatment where systemic exposure needs to be kept at a minimum and there needs to be precise targeting.

12.2.4 Biodegradable Implants

- Biodegradable drug delivery systems can be made of polymers such as PLGA or PCL that can deliver drugs directly to a target site for weeks or even months. These applications include local cancer therapy, hormone replacement therapy, and chronic pain management.

12..3. Mechanisms of Biodegradation

There are several mechanisms of biodegradation of biodegradable drug delivery systems that depend on material composition, the body's environment, and the desired period of drug release.

- **Hydrolytic Degradation:** Most of the biodegradable polymers, like PLGA and PLA, degrade via hydrolysis. In this process, the polymer chains break due to exposure to water molecules over time, resulting in slow degradation.

- **Enzymatic Degradation:** A few biodegradable materials degrade on the action of specific enzymes. Chitosan and collagen hydrogels are degraded naturally by the body's own enzymes; therefore, they are great for tissue engineering and wound healing.

- **pH-Responsive Degradation:** Acidity-driven systems, developed for such acidic environments, as in tumor sites, would employ materials that degrade much faster at lower pH values and thus release the drug payload more effectively in target areas.

12.4 Medical Applications of Biodegradable Systems

Biodegradable systems are multidisciplinary, and various applications have been reported in the fields of medicine. Some of these most impactful applications include;

- **Medicine Localized Chemotherapy:** Biodegradable implants containing the chemotherapeutic agents that can be implanted close to the tumors, thus locally delivering drugs to the targeted cancer cells and reducing its systemic side effects. This treatment is already in practice by implanting biodegradable wafers containing drugs immediately after surgery for the treatments of brain cancers.

- **Nanoparticles targeted therapy:** Such biodegradable nanoparticles will be used as drug delivery systems with the focusing on delivering those drugs directly to cancerous cells. This would allow a decrease in the dosage of drugs that decreases the damage caused to the other normal tissues. Such devices can also be constructed that would only become activated, for example, in a given acidic environment, which is only present within the tumors.
- **Orthopedics and Bone Repair:** Bone Regeneration Implants: Biodegradable implants that are used in the delivery of growth factors and antibiotics to promote healing in bones. The therapeutic agents from these biodegradable implants are slowly and steadily released to induce bone regeneration without requiring the need for secondary surgery for removal of the implant.
- **Drug-Loaded Scaffolds:** Drug releasing scaffolds may be prepared from biodegradable material to deliver drugs that could improve bone repair in case of fractures and other forms of bone injuries. This scaffold also offers a structural matrix for the growth of new bone cells.
- **Wound Healing and Tissue Engineering:** Wound healing: Biodegradable hydrogels Biodegradable hydrogels maintain the moisture inside the wound and

support more rapid healing; along with the ability to incorporate the antibiotics to prevent the secondary infection. There is no dress removal hassle in biodegradable hydrogels as it resorbs if healing is continued by definition.

- **Skin and Tissue Regeneration:** Most tissue engineering uses biodegradable polymers to create scaffolds to support cell growth and tissue formation. At the end of healing, the scaffold degrades, leaving behind all-natural tissue.
- **Biodegradable Stents:** Biodegradable stents are offered in order to stabilize the arteries after surgical intervention until it can work alone without having to support it. Once provided, these biodegradable stents melt over time; such have less risk in the long-term since they will melt.
- **Drug-Eluting Stents:** These are used for drug-eluting stents which prevent the restenosis of arteries and most are made from biodegradable polymers as they elute anti-inflammatory or anti-proliferative drugs at a slow release.

- **Ophthalmology:** Biodegradable Ocular Inserts: Implants that can administer drugs for a prolonged period are used in the management of chronic eye diseases including macular edema and glaucoma. In this case, using a biodegradable implant at least injections are avoided, thus improving patient comfort and compliance.

12.5 Case Studies: Successful Biodegradable Drug Delivery Systems:

- **Gliadel Wafer in Brain Cancer:** Gliadel is a biodegradable implant that contains a chemotherapeutic agent named carmustine. After the tumors are removed through surgery, these wafers implanted in the brain slowly begin to release a drug targeting residual cancerous cells within the brain tissue. As a localized form of delivering drugs, gliadel reduces the systemic exposure as it promotes higher concentrations at the point of the tumor.

- **Hormone Therapy Zoladex® Implant:** A biodegradable implant where the hormone goserelin is released to be given for prostate and breast cancer patients. A slower release of a drug will mean fewer side effects will occur. Since it's a biodegradable preparation, surgical removal of an implant will not be needed.

- **Ozurdex is a biodegradable ocular implant:** The implant was devised for the administration of dexamethasone ocular treatment for macular edema. As can be observed, it permits steady release of the drug dexamethasone without the need for multiple injections into the eyes that will directly act to reduce inflammation or improve vision.

12.6 Future Outlooks: A Promising Future For Drug-Delivery Systems

Future prospects indicate that research in biodegradable drug delivery systems holds brilliant promises: they emphasize more precision, better outcomes, and sustainability of the product.

- **Smart Biodegradable Systems:** Scientists have created biodegradable systems that are responsive to specific physiological conditions, such as temperature, pH, or the presence of specific enzymes. Such systems deliver drugs only when required, thus maximising therapeutic effects while minimising the potential side effects.

- **Multi functional biodegradable material:** Advances in the area of materials science would enable for the first time in nature the design of biodegradable systems that could serve more than one function. Such an application would include delivery of drug with structural support. Even now, it is well within our imagination to picture design of scaffolds of growth factor that promotes the regeneration of bone while eliminating infection.

- **Biochemical sensors:** Some potential interactions of the biodegradable drug delivery system with wearable technology are real-time monitoring and adjustment of drugs within the body. Biochemical sensors within wearable technologies monitor biomarkers within the body to deliver a signal to a biodegradable device, thereby regulating medication and ensuring proper treatment.

- **Environmental Sustainability:** The new study now has added cellulose-based polymers as a dimension that includes the natural source with which the system might find renewal once applied to biodegradable systems, hence bringing less bad influence to the environment. That said, further advancement paves the way to spark further interest in health-care technology about sustainability.

Conclusion: Biodegradable drug delivery systems point toward the future of medicine. Patients would then be under care, but it also pays off to be environmentally responsive. The foregoing will then be of a different kind because these will effectively eliminate the need to have devices removed, cut environmental burdens, and afford control over local drug delivery. Hence, it would involve applications by biodegradable drug delivery systems in new roles meant for chronic and complicated disease management and provide much more innovative and sustainable solution models. Controlled-Release Systems would be taken as the next chapter that focuses on the furtherance of therapeutic outcomes in modern medicine.

Chapter 13: Gene Therapy And Viral Vectors: Innovative Drug Delivery Solutions

Gene therapy is, without a doubt, one of the most promising disciplines within modern medicine. It allows for the treatment of diseases caused by genetics, such as cancers and any disease that has proven especially resistant to traditional treatments. Unlike many traditional therapies, which address symptoms, gene therapy works on the root cause that leads to the disease-the genetic cause - perhaps the reason for successful long-term treatment or even cures. However, the basis of successful gene therapy remains one critical component: an effective and safe method for the delivery of therapeutic genes or gene-editing tools into the targeted cells. In this chapter, we explore some of the innovative drug delivery solutions developed for gene therapy, focusing on viral vectors-one of the most efficient and commonly used methods for transferring genetic material into cells.

13.1 Fundamentals of Gene Therapy

Gene therapy is an application of the principle of changing or introducing genetic material into cells in a patient to correct disease or mitigate it. There are three approaches: by replacing a faulty gene; by adding a new gene; or by editing an existing gene so that a mutation is corrected. These strategies alter cellular function at the genetic level, either to reverse aberrant activity in cells that contain defective genes or to introduce new functions into cells, such as allowing the immune system to recognize and attack cancer cells. Some of the strategies used in gene therapy include:

- **Gene Replacement Therapy:** The malfunctioning gene is replaced with a healthy copy.
- **Gene Addition Therapy:** A new gene is introduced to fight disease.
- **Gene Silencing:** This involves using RNA interference or other methods to silence a particular gene causing the disease.
- **Gene Editing:** These use CRISPR/Cas9 technologies that directly correct mutations in the DNA origin at the cell level.

13.2 Challenges to Gene Delivery

One of the biggest challenges gene therapy confronts is how to administer genetic material safely and with efficiency into the right cell. The human body also presents many barriers to protect against foreign DNA that cells contain, making it hard for therapeutic genes to reach such cells. Some of them include:

- **Cellular barriers:** The cell membrane rejects the entry of foreign objects, including therapeutic DNA and RNA.
- **Immune Responses:** The immune system can recognize foreign DNA and delivery vectors. This leads to the possibility of eliciting an inflammatory reaction or rejection of the vectors.

- **Target Specificity:** One of the most important attributes is getting the right gene to reach only the diseased cells that are affected sparing normal cells both for efficacy as well as safety.
- **Stability:** Genetic material is fragile, and it is degradable, so a robust delivery system will be crucial to protecting therapeutic genes to the target site.

Researchers have developed several delivery strategies to overcome these challenges. In clinic, viral vectors are used most efficaciously among them.

13.3 Viral Vectors in Gene Therapy

Viruses are often engineered to harbor therapeutic genes rather than the normal pathogenic material. Being capable of naturally entering cells and delivering genetic material, viruses are efficient carriers, or "vectors," to use in gene therapy. The genetic material of the virus is altered so that it no longer causes disease but can still allow infection to cells with therapeutic DNA or RNA. Most frequently used viral vectors in gene therapy include:

- **Adenovirus Vectors:** These vectors create strong immunity and are applied in applications where high levels of gene expression are needed over a short period. They are mainly applied in cancer therapy and vaccine application but may induce an immune response.
- **Adeno-Associated Virus (AAV) Vectors :** The AAV is considered non-pathogenic; it can even undergo genomic integration into the host genome, giving a great

edge for long-term expression in gene therapy. So, in this regard, AAV vectors have widely been employed for the treatment of some genetic disorders such as spinal muscular atrophy and some types of inherited forms of blindness.

- **Lentivirus Vectors:** These are based on HIV and can integrate into the host cell genome, enabling long-term expression. They are widely used in CAR-T cell therapies, in which a patient's immune cells are genetically engineered to recognize and attack cancer cells.
- **Retrovirus Vectors:** Retroviruses share all properties of lentiviruses except that they insert themselves into the host genome. While other viruses infect all body cells, retroviruses only enter the cells that are dividing in culture. This places an important limitation on use in treatment of disease as it can only target locations in the body where dividing cells exist. The good examples of such diseases treated include blood diseases.

Advantages and Limitations of Viral Vectors

There are numerous reasons why viral vectors, especially due to their effectiveness of gene transfer, become convenient tools for gene therapy. The following are notable among them:

- **Highly efficient:** Viral vectors carry genetic material to cells and enter them efficiently to achieve a desired therapeutic outcome.
- **Cell type-targeting:** The viral vector has the potential to be targeted to certain types of cells, thereby ensuring

that off-target effects are minimized by increasing the accuracy of drug delivery.

Viral vector can carry large genes, therefore it can integrate permanently and deliver long-term gene expression which is useful in chronic diseases and a great advantage in viral treatment.

Limitations:
- It elicits some type of immune response from hosts which is especially noticed using an adenovirus. The therapeutic use of it to certain chronic diseases and application gets a little restricted thereby.
- Viral vectors are limited in their cargo carrying capacity, so they could only carry a limited amount of DNA, which is very restricting for large genes.
- **Insertional Mutagenesis:** The possibility that integrated viral vectors might interfere with the normal function of host genes is a potential hazard and may contribute to cancer, which is particularly the case with the use of retrovirus and lentivirus vectors.

13.5 Alternatives to Non-Viral Gene Delivery

While viral vectors are the most efficient tool for gene delivery known thus far, non-viral delivery methods have recently dealt with many of the problems associated with viral vectors including immune response and size constraint for cargo. Among such methods are:

- **Liposomes and Lipid Nanoparticles:** DNA or RNA can be entrapped within lipid-based nanoparticles to make it non-degradable by enzymes, thus making it cell-permeable. mRNA vaccines against COVID-19 employ the use of this technology while promising more use in gene delivery.
- **Polymeric Nanoparticles:** The PLGA biodegradable polymer may be designed to provide slow release of genetic material, thus potentially reducing immune response while targeted delivery can still be achieved.
- **Electroporation:** In this, electrical pulses temporarily open pores in cell membranes which allow the genetic material to be allowed inside. This method is conducted in gene therapy research though not so practical in the clinic because it is an invasive technique.
- **Gene Guns:** These are machines that "fire" microscopic particles coated with DNA into cells. Application of this method is mostly in research and experimental gene therapy for localised treatments.

13.6 Applications of Gene Therapy and Viral Vectors: Gene therapy with the help of viral vectors has become a very promising drug for the treatment of numerous diseases. The most important applications are:

- The treatment of a genetic disorder such as SMA, wherein functional copies of the mutated gene are delivered into patient cells using AAV vectors.
- The other is the targeted delivery of the gene to treat the inherited blindness called Leber's congenital amaurosis.

- It was a revolution with viral vectors, especially lentivirus-based CAR-T therapies, transforming the way cancer is currently being treated. The CAR-T therapy is a mode of therapy where the T-cells of the patient are engineered to recognize a specific marker of cancer so that the immune system can now identify and kill those cells. CAR-T therapy has worked well in the treatment of certain leukemias and lymphomas.
- The same case goes with neurodegenerative diseases, such as for Parkinson's or Huntington's- in those diseases, some drugs are present, though the levels of efficacy are too low.
- Gene therapy involves the viral vector-based model that treats infections. This case is very manifest in vaccines made against Covid-19 that is based on the use of adenoviral vectors to deliver a code of genetics that will initiate viral protein and provoke immune reactions without any risk of causing infections.

13.7 Ethical and Regulatory Concerns in Gene Therapy

With gene therapy progress come a new set of ethical concerns and regulations. Permanent genetic alterations include genes transmitted across generations in germline cells. Permanent alterations in the genes may have unpredictable adverse effects or serve as an avenue for causing harm. Gene therapies, especially viral vector-based ones, are known to induce an immune response and even cause genomic damage; therefore, these must be tested in the laboratory for their safety and efficacy. The FDA and EMA strictly regulate the release of gene therapies into the market.

Ethical issues also include the cost of gene therapy-many gene therapies are too expensive, which has raised issues of accessibility and equity. As the technology of gene therapy continues to advance, regulatory frameworks evolve to answer these issues so that gene therapies are safe, effective, and accessible for those who need them.

13.8 Future Directions and Innovations

Currently, studies are being conducted that seek to make gene therapy safer and more effective and easier to administer. The most prominent innovations that are going to be seen soon are:

- **Viral Vectors:** Advanced design of viral vectors reduces the immune responses, increases the capacity of cargo carrying, and also enhances targeting specificity.
- **Gene Editing:** Techniques such as CRISPR/Cas9 and prime editing make very precise gene edits and are in the phase of potential use in clinic.
- **Non-viral technologies:** These encompass continued advancements in lipid nanoparticle-based, polymeric carrier systems, as well as other forms of nonviral technologies. Such technologies appear to offer safer alternatives compared with viral vectors.
- **Personalized gene therapy:** It based on the advancement in genomics, will allow for the tailored design of gene therapies according to an individual's specific genetic profile to bring about improved outcomes.

It brings out the possible transformational power of gene therapy and viral vectors to treat what was once regarded as untreatable. Amidst all these challenges, innovation is not stopping and appropriate regulation continues to make gene therapy an increasingly viable option for a wide range of diseases, opening new possibilities in future healthcare.

Chapter 14: Regulatory Challenges In Drug Delivery System Development

The drug delivery system is one of the multidisciplinary fields that involve pharmacology, chemistry, engineering, and medicine. Emerging innovations dictate that regulatory frameworks should fit safety as well as efficiency with opportunities for innovation. In this chapter, we will reflect on the complex landscape of challenges in the development of drug delivery systems, meaning to point out key issues, processes, and the imperative towards balanced regulation.

14.1. Role of Regulatory Oversight US FDA, EMA:

Role of Regulatory Oversight US FDA, EMA, and others all over the world form an important part of the new drug delivery system's development approval process.

- They primarily act to protect public health through drugs which are safe and effective in manufacture.

- It would have to pass all the safety and effectiveness tests before hitting the market; in other words, it has to pass through a number of preclinical studies and clinical trials.

- **Prevent Harm:** Regulatory agencies work towards preventing adverse effects or harmful outcomes that may arise from the use of new drug delivery systems, including problems with toxicity, pharmacokinetics, and long-term effects.

- **Promote Innovation:** A regulatory way could push for innovation on a high scale due to having the direction and way research scientists as well as other drug developing firms navigate in arriving with something in the market.

14.2. Unique challenges to Drug delivery System

It is quite complicated than a Pharmaceutical. Here, there is the development, making a challenge. A portion of unique regulatory difficulties which accompany is;

- **Complexity of Delivery Systems:** The drug delivery system can have many constituents, which may include nanoparticles, liposomes, polymers, etc. It is likely that each of them has distinct regulatory requirements and so the interaction will make it difficult to decide on safety and efficacy.

- **Combination Products:** This class is also drug delivery systems and thus considered combination products. The class could be either a drug-device combination or biologic-drug combination. Such products may have unclear pathways for regulation because they would potentially involve review by several regulatory divisions.

- **New Technologies:** New delivery systems were discovered under the umbrella of nanotechnology, gene therapy, and biotechnology. Such new delivery systems may not fit conveniently under the existing categories of regulations and therefore may make it uncertain what of the regulations might apply or how safety and efficacy are demonstrated.

14.3. Regulatory Pathway: Overview

Critical steps through which drug delivery systems need to traverse in the regulatory pathway are as follows:

- **Preclinical Development**: At the preclinical stage, a drug delivery system must be developed so that it can be administered to humans. It would not be safe to administer to humans without first establishing that the drug delivery system is safe and may be effective. This normally involves in vitro studies within the laboratory and in vivo studies in animals. Depending on the nature of such studies, regulatory agencies will require complete documentation of the safety profile of the drug delivery system.

- **The actual first step**, after preclinical studies, will be the submission of an Investigational New Drug Application. This application includes all information from the preclinical study, a proposed plan for the clinical study, manufacturing information, and proposals for the monitoring of safety in the clinical trial period.

- **Clinical trials- done in phases:** Phase 1, 2, and 3. The checkup for the safety of the drug delivery system, efficacy, appropriate dosing, and so forth is to be done.

Regulatory agencies closely watch this, so adverse events should be evident.

- **NDA or BLA:** In case of small molecules, the developers submit an NDA, while for biologics, a BLA is submitted after the clinical trials have been successfully conducted to be granted marketing approval. It includes all data of all phases of testing, such as proposed labeling and manufacturing details.

- **Post-Market Surveillance:** Once approved, regulatory agencies require the manufacturer to continue surveillance of the safety and effectiveness of a drug delivery system. They have to report adverse events and perform post-marketing studies as required.

14.4. Specific Regulatory Issues:

Specific regulatory issues that would come up while developing drug delivery systems are:

Manufacturing and Quality Control: GMPs would have to be followed in ensuring that the drug delivery systems are manufactured consistently, thereby guaranteeing the quality and safety. There has to be stringent testing for raw materials, processes for manufacturing, and finished products. Quality control would pose considerable challenges, especially when dealing with complicated systems, more so regarding nanotechnology.

Labeling and Claims: Labeling of drug delivery systems must be accurate enough for health providers and patients to know how to properly and safely use the product. Agencies charged with regulating examine the claims of the manufacturer determining whether such claims have any evidence from scientific sources.

Risk Benefit Analysis: One major risk-benefit analysis by the regulatory agencies has to be made concerning whether the potential benefits of a drug delivery system are worth more than the risks. Such an assessment varies and can be arguably subjective between agencies, which, in this case, can lead to uncertainty in terms of the approval for the drug delivery system.

Patient Population Factors: The nature of the patient population to be targeted also plays a role in the regulatory decision. For example, drug delivery systems for targeting the pediatric or geriatric population will likely attract greater regulatory scrutiny to guarantee safety and efficacy in those populations.

14.5. How to Successfully Navigate the Regulatory Environment

Drug delivery system developers can use several strategies to successfully navigate the regulatory environment.

- ☐ **Involve regulatory authorities:** at an earlier phase so that all information before development and further feedback after any development plans are ready. Pre-

IND discussions and consultations proved helpful with clarifying the expectations set on by the regulators and make the application more streamlined as well.

☐ **Design Robust Preclinical Studies:** A well-designed preclinical study conducted according to the regulatory requirement can easily get into the clinic. It refers to the proper use of appropriate models with suitable endpoints in reflection of the clinical use.

☐ **Implement Quality by Design:** QbD is the proactive approach to product development, focusing on understanding the factors that affect quality and performance. Through the adoption of QbD principles, developers can improve consistency and reduce regulatory hurdles.

☐ **Thorough Documentation:** All studies, manufacturing processes, and quality control measures should be documented in detail. In this way, ensuring all data is well-organized and readily accessible can help make regulatory reviews and inspections smoother.

☐ **Keep Informed of Changes in Regulations:** The regulatory framework is constantly changing, particularly in the light of progress in science and technology. Developers can adjust their strategies by keeping themselves updated with changes in regulations and guidance.

14.6. Future Directions in Regulatory Science

☐ Drug delivery systems are advancing day after day, and so is the regulatory science. A few future directions may alter the landscape of regulation:

☐ Agencies can use more adaptive frameworks such that flexibility can be applied in the assessment of a new drug delivery system. For example, expedited pathways may be put forward for breakthrough technologies or adaptively designed trials to follow emerging data.

☐ The current practice is applying real-world evidence to make regulatory decisions. RWE is evidence that relies upon experience from the real world to help assess the drug delivery system in terms of effectiveness and safety after it receives approval.

☐ International Harmonization: Regulation of drug delivery systems in the various countries and regions will help obtain approval for such systems in all the world's nations. Standardization of the regulatory requirements can be considered as the effort of International Council for Harmonisation, ICH, to lessen the entry barriers.

☐ Advanced Integration of Technological Innovations: In regulation processes, AI and ML can be used in integration of their functions toward better and efficient review systems as well as risk assessments. Those technologies can help in producing predictions based on huge quantities of data while refining the sense of decision making.

Conclusion

This requires several regulatory hurdles at stages, which has to be tackled very cautiously by developers and researchers along with members who form the regulatory body. Therefore, with proper knowledge of complexities of regulatory lands and strategy for satisfying all regulatory requirements, one could help develop innovative drug delivery systems into a good stage of success. With advancement in science and the emergence of new technologies, dialogue between regulators and the pharmaceutical industry will be of paramount importance to their endeavors in ensuring that such advancements are realized in the context of safety to public health. It is determined not by the scientific advancement but by the regulatory framework that governs their development and use.

Chapter 15 Future Perspectives: Emerging Trends And Technologies In Drug Delivery

With the fast pace of drug delivery advancement, new technologies and methodologies are being developed promising to enhance efficacy, improve safety profiles, and also enhance patient compliance with therapeutic interventions. The following chapter discusses a few advanced trends and technologies emerging in this field to shape the future of drug delivery-advancements in nanotechnology, personalized medicine, smart drug delivery systems, and integration of artificial intelligence and machine learning.

15.1 Nano Technology Advances

Drug delivery systems have undergone changes through nanotechnology, making nanoscale drug carriers able to be designed with improved drug solubility and stability that increases the drug bioavailability. They can target particular tissues and cells so as not to affect any others unnecessarily while increasing the potential for beneficial results from treatment.

- **Nanoparticles and Nanocarriers:** These include liposomes, dendrimers, polymeric nanoparticles which encapsulate drugs and release these in controlled manners. For instance, preparation of nanoparticles that deliver chemotherapeutic agents directly to the malignant cells could minimize side effects more commonly associated with the treatment of cancer, and thereby spare healthy cells.

- **Responsive Nanocarriers :** The trends also include self-assembled stimuli-responsive nano-particles which can act as stimuli-sensitive drug-carriers. Such nano-devices will respond to environmentally sensitive stimuli such as pH-based, temperature-sensitive, and biomarker-based triggers leading to controlled payload release.

This technology offers a higher precision in drug delivery and allows directed therapeutic intervention.

15.2 Personalized Medicine

This trend in drug delivery is said to move toward personalized medicine, which may allow designing therapy depending upon the characteristic profile of the patient, such as genetic background, lifestyle, and disease profile.

Genomic and proteomic technologies: It will enhance the genomic sequencing that allows the advancement of the proteomics technology analysis to be permitted with a process of identifying certain biomarkers, guiding the drug and dose amount. For example, drugs use in relation to some pharmacogenomics; it would have one have medicine tailor-made for those with their genetic profiles to aid the better therapy with fewer side effects.

Personalized drug formulations: Future delivery involves making customized drug formulations for a given patient. In the context of the advancements of 3D printing, the customized drug delivery devices and forms are developed and created for optimal therapeutic outputs from drugs.

15.3 Intelligent drug delivery systems

The advance drug delivery system with smart technology would be programmed to monitor the patient in real-time, control release, and ensure optimally therapeutic levels for the patient.

- **Wearable Devices:** Wearable technology containing biosensors can monitor physiological parameters like glucose or heart rate. This is directly linked to drug delivery systems wherein dosing of medicines could be executed automatically through real-time data gathered using these devices. Chronic conditions like diabetes and hypertension shall be better managed in the most effective possible manner.

- **Programmable drug delivery systems:** Such devices may have a possibility of drug release in controlled profiles. Example of such devices is an implantable drug delivery device wherein a microchip administers a definite dose at a certain time to ensure better compliance with medication.

15.4 AI/Machine Learning Integration

The relation of AI and ML is quite rapid in the case of drug delivery system and gradually it is changing a promising site for new breakthrough in design and implementation of new drug therapies.

- **Predictive Analytics:** AI will look at large amounts of data that predict how a patient will react to many drug therapies, which, based on genetics, medical background, and lifestyle, will make the best treatment choices for more tailored and hence effective therapy.

- **Optimization in Formulation Development:** Even drug formulation development can be accelerated by machine learning due to the stability and efficacy predictions the new compound would provide by using history data. This will reduce time and costs in drug development, hence quicker paths of research toward clinical applications.

15.5 Role of the Regulator

Of course, any new drug delivery technology will require assurance of safety and efficacy. The regulatory concern in keeping up with the pace of technological development is actually a patient-safety issue. For example, FDA and EMA, among all other regulatory agencies, have some policies guiding reviews on new drug delivery technologies, such as nanotechnology-based products in this case. Such policies, therefore, obviously assist developers to ensure the therapy emerging will undergo all standards of safety and efficacy.

Real-World Evidence: RWE is slowly but surely becoming an integral part of the regulation assessment of new drug delivery systems. It may provide an avenue toward understanding how the new therapies work in everyday real-life clinical settings complementing the data obtained from clinical studies.

15.6 Future Challenges and Considerations

A lot more challenging challenges await to actually realize the promise of emerging technologies.

- The possibility of personalizing medicine, as it involves consequences with the feasibility of medical care and side effects because of genetic testing, brings along ethical issues. It, therefore, calls for consideration to such issues when ensuring that all patients benefit equally in drug delivery technology.

- Cost and Accessibility: The most recent developed drug delivery systems might be even more expensive to develop and make, and therefore accessible populations of patients might be limited. If these gains are going to benefit large number, these cost barriers shall need to be overcome over the coming years.

- The scientific world too also brings with it the burden of continually assessing its long-term safety and efficacy.

- Continuous monitoring and post-marketing surveillance will be the safeguard to patients and the efficiency to new therapies.

Conclusion

The fast advancement of drug delivery is sure a promising breakthrough in outcomes related to patients. Scientists and healthcare professionals are on their way to these recent inventions in nanotechnology, customized medication, smart systems, and AI in the management of the new and more patient-focusing therapies. But, as the area of advancement continues to unfold, there is no doubt that this will force some of these challenges into its face for its requirement and guarantee that not only are they safe but also accessible. It's beyond doubt, as the future and further definition of drug delivery is shaped by an inevitable act of modern medicine, collaboration among the researchers, regulators, and healthcare providers.

www.ingramcontent.com/pod-product-compliance
Lightning Source LLC
Chambersburg PA
CBHW082110220526
45472CB00009B/2122